BIOCHROMY

BIOCHROMY

Natural Coloration of Living Things

Denis L. Fox

UNIVERSITY OF CALIFORNIA PRESS

Berkeley   Los Angeles   London

University of California Press
Berkeley and Los Angeles, California

University of California Press, Ltd.
London, England

Printed in the United States of America

1 2 3 4 5 6 7 8 9

For Miriam and our family: Ron, Kathy, and Alan

And in loving memory of Steve (1935-1954)

Biochromy: Natural Coloration of Living Things

by Denis L. Fox

ERRATA

Page 8, line 27: *for* "stripe" *read* "stipe"

Page 31, line 12: *for* "and" *read* "or"

Page 39, line 27: *between* "only" *and* "carotenoid" *insert* "or preponderant"

Page 51, line 16: *add* comma after "surprisingly" *and delete* comma after "detected"

Page 56, line 11: *after* semicolon *read* "here are present carotenes"

Page 130, line 11: *delete* "a" *before* "vitamin B_{12}"

Page 148, line 22: *for* "methyl" *read* "acetic"

Page 151, line 30: *for* "Actiniochematin" *read* "Actiniohematin"

Page 159, line 13: *for* "vevers" *read* "Vevers

Page 189, lines 27 and 28: *for* "CU" *read* "Cu"

In Index under *Limulus polyphemus*: *for* "hemoglobin" read *"hemocyanin"*

Contents

Preface

You who explore this book probably belong, together with its author, to a community of persons who share an abiding love for living nature. Plants and animals may claim our attention owing to many different aspects, whether comparative size and shape; means of growth, movement, and adaptation; economic importance; or simply the sheer, contrasting beauty of color and pattern. In the words of the botanical chemist Michael Tswett, "Our minds seem naturally inclined to devote special attention to all coloured substances." It was this latter condition of nature that in large part prompted the book's title *Biochromy,* from *bios* [Gk., "life"] and *chroma* [Gk., "color"].

The great variety of colors in our natural surroundings has doubtless attracted the admiration, wonder, and searching curiosity of humans since the emergence of our species. This applies especially to color manifestations in living entities, which may vary as they grow, move, reproduce, or react to stimuli. Moreover, the pigmentation of living things may offer various clues of practical usefulness to the physician, the farmer or horticulturist, those involved in animal husbandry and genetics, as well as others who may need to apply colors to techniques of camouflage or industrial operations.

Much has been written, some of it dating back beyond a century, on both the popular and technical features of biological coloration, and upon the theoretical value of advertising or concealing pigmentation, as well as the usefulness of sexual dichromatism, wherein the sexes of a given species may be differently colored. Many species may exhibit one or more of these attributes. I have undertaken a considerable number of research articles, major reviews, contributing chapters, and encyclopedia entries, as well as two editions of the book *Animal Biochromes and Structural Colours.*

I should have to confess, however, that my past writings on the overall subject (beyond encyclopedic entries) have been addressed primarily to biochemists, physiologists, and general biologists, and to chemists and physicists with peripheral interests in biology. I had not earlier undertaken, as I do now, to prepare a book inviting the inquisitive general reader to partake of discussions featuring the role of prominent colors in living organisms, as well as any special physiological significance that colored chemical molecules may possess in the living economy of plants and animals.

Considering the continued accessibility of the second edition of my above-named book, published by the University of California Press in 1976, and in view of the ready availability of several other books dealing with natural pigments, I have decided that, rather than citing extensive numbers of original sources, reference to broader treatments as well as comprehensive reviews and surveys should suffice most readers. General review references therefore replace much of the usual comprehensive bibliography in this treatment of natural biochromy, addressed hopefully as it is to a wider audience. Consultation of specific original reports, listed among the secondary references cited, should serve to guide the intrepid reader farther into selected realms of more specialized inquiry.

In addressing discussions transcending so wide a field of study to an audience composed of perhaps highly diversified backgrounds and primary interests, it is inevitable that the author shall fall short of giving full satisfaction to everyone. The use of certain essential technical explanatory terms and references is unavoidable; they will be desirable to some readers and not to others.

When biochemical names must be used, I have tried to add either a passing definition or an equivalent term, or to refer to the illustrative appendix consisting of seriatim families of structural formulas, in the hope that this way of presentation may satisfy most members of my patient audience.

I owe thanks to more friends, colleagues, and students than I can name, for their respective parts in encouraging me to attempt this treatment of living coloration. Both they and I can recall in great part the ways in which I received their help. I must include specifically, however, reference to staff members of two outstanding presses: Cambridge University Press, publishers of the first, and the University of California Press, producers of the second, edition of *Animal Biochromes*. And in the case of the latter organization, publisher of the present work, I owe particular thanks to my good friends August Frugé and Robert Y. Zachary. Both of these longtime friends and colleagues, among others, urged me to respond to what they recognized as a current need for a popularized treatment of the subject.

For the color plates I am indebted to a number of people. James Lance generously supplied the photographs of the highly pigmented nudibranch slugs, and furnished their names. Edvard Hemmingsen permitted photographic reproduction of his photos of the Antarctic icefish and its colorless blood. The pictures of various fishes and invertebrates are from the collection of the Scripps Institution of Oceanography, thanks to Pat Kampmann, Larry Ford, George Koscho, and others on the staff of the aquarium and museum. Finally, most of the colored illustrations of birds and mammals were made available by the photographic department of the Zoological Society of San Diego, notably through Ron Garrison. Carl Hubbs and Richard Rosenblatt kindly named or confirmed the names of a number of fishes shown in certain photographs.

Several former doctoral students, notably half a dozen who wrote their dissertations about biochromes, receive passing identification during the treatment of appropriate subject matter. Readers thus will recognize the importance of student contributions to the forefront of our knowledge in this field of inquiry.

Prominent among those of my quondam students who co-authored papers with me, and most of whose doctoral researches are cited, include the following, in chronological sequence according to the year of their respective degrees. Their studies are also designated as to the animals or materials on which they focused: Bradley Scheer (sea mussel, 1940), Sheldon Crane (octopus, 1949), Gene Corcoran (marine sediments,

1957), Michael Pilson (abalones, 1963), George Crozier (fishes, 1967), Tom Hopkins (sea stars, 1967), Elliott Smith (sponges, 1968), Jim McBeth (nudibranch slugs, 1970), and Ned Ruby (oxygen-storing, marine beach-sand-dwelling polychaete worm, *Euzonus,* 1976).

Voluntary comments, whether from, say, a faithful laboratory helper and part-time typist, or any other source, when recognized as timely and worthy of citation, should be included and be attributed to the original author or speaker. Frequently the observation is refreshingly amusing as well as amplifying. The reader may find occasional passing references, among others, to Laughing Gull (Sioux name) or merely to her initials L-G; the name may be familiar to some who might have seen it in letters or other writings. An example: Regarding a brief reference to the Florida chameleon *Anolis carolinensis,* L-G's comment: "We call 'em politico lizards back home. From the way, you know, they change their colors according to how they feel, or to match up with their surroundings. And when they do that, and stay perfectly still, they sure can lie doggo!" Rather than insert this new, alternative, and admittedly tempting "common name" into the textual reference, I decided to preclude disappointment, and perhaps even compliment the source of suggestion, by placing the comment here.

Such a candid volunteer may sometimes emerge as master (or mistress) of the brief rejoinder. In an exchange of ideas regarding the color of an invertebrate's skin, and of the pigment's hue after extraction into various organic solvents, I was reminded of a word of advice accorded a class in advanced organic chemistry, wherein I was enrolled as an undergraduate in a long-past year. Professor T. D. Stewart said something to this effect: "I've called this dye red, as a generalizing term, but have heard any number of specific alternative hues mentioned in describing such colors. And I remind you: Never argue with a woman about a color!" So, on my having called our sea star simply a red specimen, there arose at once some alternative suggestion, supposedly a more discriminating term—whether cerise, crimson, scarlet, vermilion, madder, or what, I do not remember (not that it matters). I replied that my color terms were all merely general ones, usually not needing further specification in print for a report's purposes. Then, thinking I heard a further, murmuring comment about "using accurate terms when known," I tried to dismiss the matter cheerfully, asking, "Do you know how many different authorities there are on color names?" The response, soft and playful, but immediate (if somewhat wide of the mark): "One less than you think, maybe, Chief?" It is to such a finale that the simultaneous ring of one's telephone offers a welcome obbligato.

Finally, while in no sense a complete stranger to the demands inherent in writing for the general public, I have found elucidating my scientific notions to be quite demanding of my resources as to the printed word.

In my aim of optimizing what abilities I may possess, I invited a few colleagues, as well as friends on the staff of the University of California Press, to peruse such parts of the rough draft as they might desire and to accord to me the benefits of any criticism or comments they might pass along for improving or clarifying the presentation. The incorporation of certain editorial suggestions attests to my profound appreciation.

I could even stretch my acknowledgments to include one volunteer reader, who freely imparted her own ideas of syntax here and there through the whole of the narrative, in an alternative, supposedly literary style, the better to abet positive communication.

Always one to accord credit for earnest effort, I do so here and now, just as I have freely cited her words elsewhere. It was necessary at times, however, to point out distinctions between clear, simply written, serious English, on the one hand, and, on the other, breezy, rather chatty vernacular delivery, an area of communication wherein the young helper was at her best (and, as it all turned out, almost her only).

Again, to any and all readers who have been of help: Thank you, once more. All of you know that a work such as this owes much to the cooperation of others, and that any residual errors or other faults remain mine alone.

Scripps Institution of Oceanography   D. L. F.
University of California, San Diego

Tell me, ye knowing and discerning few,
Where I may find those seekers of the True,
Who will give heed while I my search express,
And then their goals in common most address.

(Adapted, with modification, from
a quatrain sewn into a sampler by one
Theadotia Hook, of Melksham, in 1801)

Introduction

Nature guards with stubborn tenacity many more secrets than ever may be revealed through even the most diligent research. Armed with the most sophisticated instruments and methods so far evolved, we have been able to recover relatively few refineables, from but limited veins or excavations of nature's vast stores. It amounts to no more than an axiomatic truism to remind ourselves that there are greater numbers of different proteins, for example, than there are living species of plants and animals characterized by such compounds. No two species carry the same protein, and each species, moreover, contains a number of different protein compounds. Proteins constitute the very basis of interspecific differences and variations among living organisms. But when we turn our attention to the class of naturally colored molecules which impart their chromatic properties to living systems, we come to realize that, despite the seemingly great diversity of colors and patterns exhibited, the responsible compounds are few indeed when compared to the vast numbers of living things that exhibit them. The colored classes of substances which characterize living organisms are relatively few in total numbers. There simply are not enough colored molecular species to go around. The more common important examples scarcely exceed a dozen different classes. Thus the same sources of coloration are common to countless different species. Many species therefore share an ability to synthesize such molecules or, alternatively, may actually share the molecules through their consumption of plants, or preying on other animals, or ingesting detrital substances in the wastes or dead bodies of plants and animals.

Of the color-producing bodies to be reviewed, our concern

will be primarily with those several classes which are most conspicuous, and which may serve some vital metabolic role in the economy of the carrier.

It is important, in the first place, to recall that color is displayed by organisms in two completely different ways: (1) chemically, through naturally occurring pigmentary molecules, referred to as true *biochromes,* which absorb some, while reflecting and/or transmitting other, fractions of visible light; and (2) physically, by colorless particles or structures of ultramicroscopic dimensions, affording colors called *schemochromes* [Gk. *schema,* "form"]. Such color sources are exemplified by (1) very numerous, colorless, randomly scattered, light-diffracting submicroscopic bodies which give rise to the so-called Tyndall blues of scattering;* or (2) by sundry striations or ultrathin successive films or layers, which resolve incident light into its components, known as *interference* colors, Newtonian spectra, or parts thereof.

While discussing the various classes of pigmentary molecules in the appropriate chapters, I have reflected that, although some readers may well wish to be informed or reminded concerning the chemical composition and accepted molecular formulas of the compounds named, there will be others to whose reading continuity the presentation of a structural formula within the text would constitute a kind of intrusion; and that, indeed, the sprinkling of the text with such figures might even discourage some general explorers from the outset. Hence, I have elected to list numbers of the more important representative compounds with their respective formulas in an appendix, appropriately annotated. "Nature is infinite, but he who takes note of symbols will understand all things, although not altogether" (Goethe).

Why do some chemical compounds exhibit colors and others not? Answers to such a reasonable query reside in the relative disposition of valence electrons responsible for linking together the constituent chains or rings of atoms making up the whole molecule. Such valence electrons are in a state of perpetual,

---

*So named after John Tyndall, the British physicist, who discussed the scattering phenomenon in 1869, while studying the blue colors of peat smoke issuing from the chimneys of Killarney cabins.

very rapid vibrational movement in situ. In relatively small molecules, such as those of glucose, urea, or acetic acid, and even in much larger ones, likewise of a saturated character (that is, involving no unfulfilled valences), including starches, proteins, and fatty compounds, the vibrational frequencies of the electrons are maximal; whereas in certain other large organic molecules, differing from the foregoing in having an unsaturated character, that is, involving double- or even triple-bonded pairs of atoms, the vibrational frequencies of electrons in such unfulfilled valences undergo some retardation. Multiple occurrences of this kind of modification in electronic vibrational frequency between constituent atom pairs promote a degree of special vibratory motion, or *chemical resonance,* in the whole molecule.

This resonance frequency of a compound is what governs its color. A resonating molecule absorbs, due to mutual internal frictional forces, the critical fraction of incident light from the visible spectrum whose frequency matches that of the resonant molecule. The absorbed light fraction is translated into heat and the residual, unabsorbed portion of emerging light is of a complementary color. Thus, should a compound possess resonance characteristics matching, and therefore capable of absorbing by interference, only the *shortest* light waves, that is, screening out violet and part of the blue spectral regions, the compound will appear *yellow. Red* compounds, possessing somewhat longer (slower) resonance frequencies, similarly extinguish light in the blue and green wavelengths, while substances expressing *blue* or *green* colors quench light in the red and orange realms.

If all light is absorbed equally and completely, the substance appears *black,* whereas *whiteness* results from equal and complete reflection of the whole *visible* spectrum (see pl. 35). Molecular resonance frequencies in such compounds are so rapid as to cancel out light fractions in the invisible regions only.

One might draw a rough comparison with a piano wire subjected to varying degrees of tautness. Low, medium, or high notes are evoked by inducing a vibrational frequency along the whole wire, wherever plucked, depending upon the tautness imposed. Under very high stretching tension, the vibrational responses of the wire to a touch will be so short and rapid as to be inaudible as a note (thus constituting an analogy with a white compound, possessed of only ultraviolet-length frequencies).

The light fraction reflected or transmitted by a pigment system usually includes parts of all wavelengths of visible light save for the absorbed portion. Thus the commonly seen color of a compound depends upon the *dominant,* complementary wavelength emerging.

There are reasons, quite beyond the purely aesthetic appeal or the recognition feature, why natural pigmentary compounds are of special interest. First, the very fact of chemical unsaturation, basic to the phenomenon of color, as we have seen, also confers upon such a compound a markedly greater degree of chemical reactivity; whether in being merely more subject to oxidative degradation or in some other particular, such molecules generally are more labile, and thus reactive. Second, this increased chemical lability and reactivity, when occurring in a molecular species constituting part of a living system, involves, in many instances (but not all, as we shall see), biochemical and physiological attributes of direct and vital importance to the organism's metabolic economy—often its well-being and overall success.

Some such well-known biocatalysts, or compounds which facilitate or otherwise regulate important biochemical reactions, are chlorophylls (App., 54),* responsible for photosynthesis in green plants; and hemoglobins (App., 55) which combine reversibly with atmospheric oxygen in animal blood, and which, in the root nodules of certain legumes, cooperate with symbiotic *Rhizobium* bacteria, effecting the fixation of atmospheric nitrogen. There are red cytochromes and other porphyrins which govern cellular oxidations; yellow riboflavins (App., 65) involved in the vitamin B_2 complex, and certain pterins (App., 68-70), such as xanthopterin, another yellow pigment, serving as a member of the vitamin B group; and some carotenoids (App., 1-30), such as β-carotene (App., 2) which serve as precursors to vitamin A (App., 30, important in vision, growth, and mucus secretion). Moreover, independently of its

*The following reference symbols will be used throughout the text: App., 1...etc., refers to chemical formulas in the appendix. Pl. 1...etc., designates color illustrations in the midsection of the book.

vitamin precursorship, β-carotene is known to combat the ill effects of certain light-sensitizing porphyrins appearing abnormally in the blood. There are large, nitrogenous molecules, the so-called bilichromes (App., 60-64), of thirty-three or more carbon atoms, which play a photosynthetic role in some seaweeds, or exercise other photokinetic functions, such as acting as light screens or promoters of active swimming migrations. They may participate in other reactions in response to incident light, as in the case of the important phytochrome responsible for fruit-ripening, autumn coloration, leaf fall, and other physiological processes, depending on length of exposure to red and far-red light.

Thus pigmentary color, chemical resonance and reactivity, and biochemical or physiological function often are to be recognized as interlocked properties of biologically significant compounds serving as metabolic triggers and/or accelerators.

1
Tyndall-Blue Colors of Scattered Light*

True pigmentary colors remain unchanged by grinding or crushing the parent material, whereas the schemochromes, or so-called optical colors, arising from very minute physical structures, are changed, or sometimes obliterated, by physical means. Thus, for example, blue plumage such as flight feathers from a jay (*Cyanocitta*), or from a South American macaw (*Ara macao*), will exhibit black, instead of the original blue coloration, at sites having been either tightly compressed between the steel jaws of a vise or struck against an anvil with a hammer. The natural blue color is generated by Tyndall scattering, that is, the reflection of only the shortest (violet and blue) light waves, in this instance by minute, ultramicroscopic airspaces within the horny keratin-protein of the feather barbs, while the longer waves of incident light (including yellow, orange, and red) pass through the alveolar or so-called spongy structure and are absorbed by an underlayer of dark melanin pigment. Therefore, viewing incident light through the ventral surface of a blue feather affords a dark appearance, while the blue rays are reflected back into the eye of the viewer on the other side. A hammer blow squashes the tiny blue-reflecting air vesicles, thus affording a clear windowlike view onto the black melanin screen below. This destruction of the air spaces is, of course, irreversible.

A reversible way in which to blacken a blue feather is to immerse it in a foreign fluid having a light-refracting power very close to that of the feather keratin itself (ca. n = 1.5-1.6).

*Pls. 4, 5.

Such a fluid may be prepared by dissolving cresol or phenol (carbolic acid) at sufficient concentrations in alcohol. In such a medium the feather keratin becomes invisible to the eye: the fluid replaces the air in the tiny bubblets within the feather barbs, thus implementing a clear "window" between the examiner and the black melanin lining the bottom inner surfaces of the barbs. If now the blackened feather be withdrawn from the foreign fluid and leached out by immersion in fresh alcohol, the dried feather will recover its minute enclosed air spaces and exhibit again the Tyndall-blue color of scattered light.

Blue colors of the same basic origin are evoked with equally striking effect by other biological systems, such as in areas of skin over parts of the neck and face of domestic turkey-cocks, or the double-wattled cassowary, *Casuarius galateus,* the skin covering the tails of certain lizards, such as the blue-tailed skink, *Eumeces skiltonianus,* and the integument characterizing the sides of the muzzle or covering parts of the haunches or buttocks and genital regions of some baboons, such as the West African mandrill *Mandrillus sphinx,* and other primates. Blue eyes, for example, of humans, Siamese cats, and nilgai antelope (the latter reportedly blue-green), offer other examples wherein a pigment-free (or very pale yellow) iris overlies the dark uveal membrane. In all such examples, the light-scattering particles are, of course, not air, as in the lifeless feather-barb structure, but small, refracting, ultramicroscopic entities, whether composed of protein, fatty substances, or both, suspended in otherwise very clear tissue overlying deeper layers (e.g., of dermal skin, pls. 4, 5), bearing heavy deposits of dark pigment.

It is important to realize that the manifestation of blue-scattering is a phenomenon depending upon the critically *small sizes* of the responsible microbodies. Their diameters or other dimensions lie in ranges around 400 or 500 nm at the most, a nanometer (nm) being equal to one-millionth of a millimeter or about one four-hundred-millionth of an inch.

WHITENESS

Feathers wherein micro air vesicles exceed about 700 nm in diameter within the barbs are white, for the same reason as with white fur or hair; the incident light is scattered reflectively, equally, and completely. Similarly, when colloidally or other very finely dispersed particulate solids or fluids in skin tissues exceed the critical diameter of 700 nm, the tissue appears white or some very light hue. It may be somewhat pink due to the presence of small capillary blood vessels; or black or other dark hues of melanin may be evident in the epidermis; even yellow, orange, or red colors may be present, due, for example, to carotenoid pigments, which will be discussed in another chapter.

It is of interest that certain feathers and hair owe their whiteness to the same fundamental condition, that is, the presence, within the dry keratin-protein, or multiple air spaces exceeding the critical size productive of blue scattering; that, nevertheless, while feathers may contain in their barbs air vesicles small enough to selectively reflect the blue and violet Tyndall colors, there are no instances of *naturally* blue hair,* that is, arising from the same microstructures. The melanin pigment of the core, or medulla, in the center of a hair is gradually replaced by a solid froth or pith, wherein the air spaces are too large to reflect any save all-white light.

Whiteness in skin or other tissues may be encountered commonly among many vertebrates and invertebrates, for example, the snow-white skin of the narwhal, the ventral skin of the killer whale (pl. 35) and bodies of some anemones, e.g., *Metridium* (pl. 27), to name a few, as well as various plants, for example, birch or aspen with their white bark; in fungi with white surfaces over the pileus or cap, or covering the stripe (stem); in aerenchymous (air-laden) tissues of some blossoms; and in the interiors of freshly cut fruits, such as apples or pears, or of potato tubers. When cut, such exposed surfaces soon darken, through ruddy, yellow-brown, and deeper colors as melanin pigment is generated from exposure to atmospheric oxygen (see below).

There are few if any known instances of Tyndall-blue light-scattering in the tissues of plants. Whereas the blues of many animal tissues arise, as we have seen, from Tyndall scattering,

---

*The questionable attractiveness of blue hair is evoked chemically by some persons, rather than occurring "Tyndally." L-G.

there are blue pigments (which will be dealt with later) in the form of plant anthocyans, or certain carotenoid pigments conjugated with protein, as in certain colorful marine invertebrates.

But there is a nonbiological phenomenon of blue-scattering, apart from the Tyndall source, from reflection by ultrafine particles; this is the so-called Rayleigh scattering, effected through very thick layers of ordinarily transparent molecules. Blue skies afford the commonest example; there the thick layers of air molecules afford the reflected blue light. At heights above the atmospheric layer, the view is black. Pure water affords another example of such scattering of blue rays; when a source of white light, whether direct or reflected, is viewed from considerable depth in very clear water, the color observed is blue. The same is true if one looks through a column of another fluid, such as ether, illuminated through a lens or pinhole-sized side window in the tube; the soft-blue cone of scattered crossing light can be viewed through a lens at the end of the containing tube.

Again, referring to seawater masses, these, when relatively near shore, may contain large populations of yellowish-colored, single-celled plant or animal species. As a consequence, not typical Rayleigh blue colors, but complementary greenish hues are seen, from the reflection (or transmission) of the yellow pigmentary colors along with the blue of scattering.

Similarly, the green iris color of some human and other animal eyes arises from the reflected scattering of Tyndall blue light plus the reflection of the light-yellowish or pale yellow-brown colors of certain melanic pigments suspended in the stroma of the iris. With increasingly larger amounts of iris melanin, the reflected color deepens from dark green to tawny or light brown, to darker browns, and finally black. Albinos' eyes show pink coloration of the iris due to the absence of pigment, such as in an underlying uveal membrane, and the consequent view of hemoglobin in the blood capillaries visible through the transparent "window." Some albino eyes may be very pale purplish colored, due to minor Tyndall scattering combined with the reflected color of hemoglobin.

True Tyndall scattering results from specific reflection of only the short violet and blue light waves as these encounter minute particles of sizes closely approximating the critical wavelength dimensions. These are reflected back, while the longer light waves pass through and are absorbed by the underlying dark screen. This blue-scattering can be demonstrated experimentally with a cubelet or preferably a small, short cylinder of agar-gel or gelatin, Light seen *through* such an object has a pale, rather dirty-yellowish color; yet when placed on a black surface and regarded in a side view or from above, the gel manifests a blue color. If then stained a pale yellow, for example, by brief immersion in an aqueous chromate solution, and replaced on the dark surface, the block of gel shows a green, often a grass-green, color.

We have seen that two sources of color evocation may act in unison to produce a new color. The green colors of some (but not all) feathers arise from the manifestation of Tyndall blue plus cuticular pigmentary *yellow* reflected light, while purple hues result from blue scattering coincident with reflection of a *red* color from the feather cuticle. The green colors in some insect bodies (again, not all) and in the skin of some reptiles, amphibians, and fishes may arise from similar, coincidentally acting sources of blue and yellow. Areas of purple coloration may be seen situated contiguously to both the blue-scattering and the richly vasculated, red regions of skin, whether covering the face and neck of cassowaries (pl. 4) and turkeys, or characterizing the muzzle, haunches, and sexual parts of baboons and some other primates. The blue or bluish sacral or so-called Mongolian patches of skin observed on or near the buttocks of some newly born infants of oriental ancestry owe their color to light-scattering within the white skin tissues overlying black deposits of melanin in the corium or dermal layer below.

Certain dyschromias, or abnormal pigmentary colorations, such as "birthmarks," sometimes called "port-wine" blemishes of human skin, owe their appearance, as in some instances cited above, to the superimposed effects of the red colors of hemoglobin and Tyndall scattering of blue light over melanin-pigmented areas in the dermis below. Cessation of circulation, with drainage of blood from the capillaries, following the person's death, confers upon a quondam purple nevus a bluish or blue-gray appearance, from the effects of light-scattering alone.

2
Colors Arising from Interference

The other principal schemochromic examples applying to living systems are encountered in many animals, and there are a few examples among plants. These include the Newtonian colors arising from interference between entering waves of incident light and returning waves, reflected from multiple inner surfaces of successively lower strata of material.

INTERFERENCE COLORS
(pls. 1-3, 14)

All observers are quite familiar with the Newtonian spectra of schemochromes, as seen, for example, from oil films on a dark, wet pavement; in the feathers of many birds, such as peafowl, hummingbirds, and mallard drakes; in bodies, wings, or wing covers (elytra) of many insect species; in genuine pearl, or in the shell nacre or so-called mother-of-pearl, encountered among certain molluscs, such as the pearl oyster and abalone (pl. 1).

The basic principle underlying the manifestation of interference colors was first discussed by Sir Isaac Newton, in his *Opticks,* first published in 1704. It was later further explained by the senior and younger Lords Rayleigh, British physicists whose writings on the subject appeared between the years 1919 and 1923.

Unlike the diffraction of direct beams of incident light into its bright spectral components, such as afforded by extremely fine gratings or striae (see below), the colors manifested by interference, through asynchrony between the component wavelengths of entering and returning light, can occur under indirect or diffused light, for example, within a room.

Interference-color manifestation depends on the presence of ultrathin alternating films of layers of different materials, whose submicroscopic dimensions match, or often may be even shorter than, the λ (wavelength) of visible light, some materials involving thicknesses as low as 50 to 150 nm. Pearl and nacre were cited above, presenting an instance wherein the alternating submicrolayers are constituted of calcium carbonate and water. The resultant colors change as the viewer alters the angle of vision. If pearl or nacre is allowed to become desiccated, that is, if, for example, all the enclosed water films should be expelled by heat, the material assumes a "dead," irreversible, matte-white appearance, whole incident light now being reflected. It is for such reason that true pearls are worn advisedly next to the skin, which is always slightly moist, and therefore affords enough water vapor to offset any tendency to evaporation of the water films within the pearl substance.*

Newtonian iridescence colors are readily demonstrable experimentally. Two simple ways may be cited. In one procedure, soapy water, with a little glycerol added, is gently shaken in a closed glass container to produce large bubbles and cusps. If then a particularly large bubble cusp is selected, and the container rotated to afford a position rendering the cusp perpendicular to the table, there will soon appear a complete set of horizontal color bands, in the following downward sequence as observed and classified by Newton (in *Opticks,* 1730):

1. Black, blue, (white), yellow, red. (Thinnest part of film at top.)
2. Violet, blue, green, yellow, red.
3. Purple, blue, green, yellow, red.

*Ladies who elect to wear a synthetic replica while keeping the true pearls in a safe or other relatively dry place would do well to heed the advice before discovering a lessened degree of iridescence manifested by a set of pearls held for a protracted sojourn in storage. The original nacreous iridescence in an abalone shell (*Haliotis rufescens*) showed no recovery after having served on the author's desk for some years as an ash tray, and often as a recipient for hot pipe dottles. L-G.

4. Green, red.
5. Greenish-blue red.
6. (Pale) greenish-blue, pale red.
7. Pale greenish-blue, reddish-white. (Least thin area at bottom.)

The very top of the settled film, being thinnest, fails to reflect light, hence remains black, while at the bottom, where the water film is thickest, the viewer perceives the palest color manifestations.

A ready manner in which to prepare a permanent display of Newtonian spectral colors is to stack a few clean glass microscope slides, the bottom member preferably blackened on its lower surface, holding the complete set between the *padded* jaws of a small laboratory screw clamp. Tightening the clamp jaws will evoke a series of spectral colors, originating from the region of highest pressure, just alongside the jaws, and spreading outward in wavy outlines. As the layers of air between the glass plates are rendered thinner by increasing pressure between the jaws of the clamp, the colored bands increase in numbers and in sharpness of definition. As with the light-scattering air vesicles in a blue feather, introduction of a fluid of the same refractive power as that of glass (in this instance) will quench all color manifestation, since the system, now rendered optically homogeneous to light, no longer displays interference.

Iridescent coloration is encountered in considerable numbers of animal species, distributed among several different phyla, and in a few plant species, to be named below. We have noted that inorganic systems such as molluscan pearls or nacre, involving alternating submicrolayers of calcium carbonate and water, present outstanding examples. Other instances are met within the hard, chitinous armor of certain crustaceans and insects; or protein materials, notably the keratins of bird feathers, scales of fishes and of reptiles, even the shed, translucent outer skin of snakes, and horny substances making up mammalian hair or nails. Indeed, even human hair, covered individually with countless minute scales, thus gains attractive luster, and shows sparkling interference colors in bright light. The so-called sea mouse *Aphrodite,* actually a large marine polychaete

worm, affords a strikingly conspicuous example of light interference from its thickly numerous, coarse, and brilliantly colored bristles.

The changeable interference colors of bird feathers are
evoked through the presence of thin, successive laminations of
different kinds or differently structured or oriented keratin proteins in the makeup of the fine barbules. The same may be said
of the brilliant schemochromes of certain insect outer cover-
ings, notably among the blue-bodied flies and wasps, and applying especially to the hard elytra of many beetles.

Among such examples, notably in beetles' elytra, as well as in
certain bird plumage, such as covers the head and neck of the
mallard drake, we encounter examples of singly predominant
coloration, whether blue, green, even gold, silvery, or other colors. These change with the angle of incidence and depend upon
the relative thickness of laminar and interlaminar layers of
material.

In an experimental setup, for example, an imitative series of a
dozen plates of transparent material having a refractive index of
1.5 may be varied as to laminar thickness and interlaminar
spaces, and observed to yield such dominant colors as in the
accompanying table.

Adding a fluid of refractive index (n) of 1.5, or very close
thereto, extinguishes the iridescent colors as the fluid enters the
interlaminar spaces.

In the case of iridescent insects and the similarly colorful
feathers of birds, air does not constitute the alternating film of
interlaminar material (save in a few instances such as *Morpho*
butterfly wing scales, cited below), but rather the chitin layers
of elytra and the keratin laminae of feathers alternate with some
other material, perhaps proteinaceous, of different refractive
index. If such materials are induced to swell, by immersion in
certain translucent fluids, the predominent interference color
undergoes a change to a longer wavelength, for example, from
initial blue to green, or even brassy. The color changes are reversible on discharge of the swelling agent, and also by applying
high, uniform pressure, which renders the structures thinner.

Colors evoked by the thin laminations of certain scarab
beetles' elytra are of considerable permanence, some having
endured in inlaid decorations within the very dry atmospheres

Thickness of each plate (nm)	Distance between plates (nm)	Angle of incidence	λ (wavelength) maximally reflected (nm)	Predominant color
50	150	60°	405	Violet
		90°	454	Blue-violet
100	100	60°	464	Blue
		90°	506	Blue-green
150	50	60°	520	Green
		90°	559	Yellow-green

in ancient Egyptian tombs. And there are far more ancient examples in nature, one instance being a large, spectrally colorful fragment of a fossil ammonite shell (a primitive nautiloid cephalopod mollusc) from a Cretaceous deposit (aged 60 to 100 million years) in a high local cliff, whence it was recovered and presented to the author by Professor Wheeler J. North while a doctoral student a quarter of a century ago.

There are beetles whose elytra exhibit red or orange schemochromic colors instead of the far commoner blue or green dominant hues. These colors of longer wavelength arise from the relatively thick laminations. The same applies to some changeable red or coppery-colored feathers, although most such hues are not changeable and are due to the presence of carotenoid pigments (to be discussed in the following chapter). Still higher orders of laminar thickness call forth conspicuous gold colors, while actual silvery aspects result from the greatest effective laminar cross section. An inanimate example of the latter effect is in a long, tightly rolled sheet of colorless cellophane, the uniform thickness of which, combined with the relatively greater interfilm air spaces, confers upon the roll the appearance of a shining bar of steel.

The minute scales covering the wings of Lepidoptera (butterflies and moths) owe their iridescent colors to the presence of hard, dry, ultrathin films of protein, separated by air spaces of similar submicroscopic fineness. In certain species of *Urania* and similar types, pressure evokes a reversible series of color changes of the same order as seen by modifying the angle of vision of the intact scale. Swelling of the structure induced by exposure to gaseous ammonia or to phenol vapor prompts reversible chromatic changes in an opposite sequence, as described earlier. Saturation of the air spaces with a fluid having a refractive index of 1.55 (closely matching that of the intact scale) reversibly extinguishes all iridescence.

Another class of beautifully iridescent wing scales is typified by those characterizing *Morpho*, a genus of brilliantly colored South American butterflies. Viewed directly from above, the wing surface reflects a magnificent, rich blue color (pl. 2). As the angle of vision is increased by tilting the wing, the viewer witnesses a sequence of blue-green to blue-violet, and finally to reddish-purple as seen from the grazing angle, close to 90° from the perpendicular. Viewed by transmitted light, the wing shows diffuse brown coloration arising from the nether layer of melanin pigment, which, by absorbing the penetrating rays, serves to enrich the play of colors reflected from the scales. Flooding of the responsible air spaces affords an interesting series of color modifications at an increasing angle of vision, as follows:

Water ($n = 1.33$): no change.
Ethyl alcohol ($n = 1.36$): bright green, blue-green, blue-purple.
Benzene-toluene-xylene ($n = 1.50$): deep green-brown.
Carbon disulfide ($n = 1.63$): brown, from direct view of melanin layer.

When the carbon disulfide is evaporated by gently blowing across the wing's upper surface, the brilliant blue color returns.

Morpho scales are nearly plane, lying shinglelike, close to the wing surface. The outer parts of the double layer of scales are long, thin, narrow structures, bearing on the upper surface many longitudinal vanes some 2-3 μ high, in rows about 1.5-2 μ apart ($1 \mu = 0.001$ mm or 1,000 nm).

Another class of scale is found among certain beetles typified by *Entimus imperialis,* the Brazilian diamond beetle. This insect has scales that are flat and elongated, without a meshed or ribbed microstructure. An outer cuticle of about 1μ thickness covers each scale, of which the thickness is perhaps 4-6 μ and which contains multiple laminations. Upper and lower surfaces of the scale display high metallic luster, usually predominating as to blue-green, but in some variants showing yellow-green or orange colors. Again the application of pressure very effectively produces the usual series of reflected colors, progressively toward the lower orders, while swelling agents induce serial changes in the opposite (redward) direction. Immersion of a torn or cut scale in a refracting liquid of $n = 1.55$ quenches the reflected and transmitted colors, disclosing complete absence of pigment, and emphasizing the internal laminated structure because of the foreign fluid's progressive invasion at successive levels.

The integument of scaleless beetles has no internal air spaces, and commonly is resistant to penetration by liquids. Protracted immersion in certain fluids, nevertheless, induces reversible swelling, with associated changes in reflected colors, such as from blue-green to greenish-brown to brass-yellow to copper-red in the elytra of the meloid beetle *Lytta vesicatoria.*

Finally, no review of the iridescent colors of interference, however brief, should omit at least passing reference to *eye-shine,* the varied and glittering reflections elicited through nocturnal illumination of numerous animal eyes. A considerable number of mammals, birds, reptiles (notably crocodilians), and amphibian species provide examples, while invertebrate instances include crustaceans (e.g., the marine crayfish or so-called spiny lobster (*Panulirus interruptus*), molluscs (*Pecten circularis,* the scallop which bears brilliant multiple polychromic eyes along the edges of its mantle), arachnids, including spiders, and many insect species.

Among the vertebrates, light is reflected from complex, striated surfaces of pigment-free materials situated deep within the eye. Predominating colors observed may be blue-green, green, yellow (or golden), red, or various serial combinations of these; they are generated by interference, and undergo considerable variation, depending on the quality of incident light, changes in the animal's pupillary aperture, or in the orientation of the viewer or of the eye itself, affecting the angle of incidence; and on fluctuations in relative quantities of blood pigments or other colored materials in the system. Differences in the predominant emerging colors, as viewed from the vertical angle, arise chiefly from the relative submicroscopic dimensions of the reflecting laminae.

In most vertebrates, responsible reflecting structures making up the *tapetum lucidum* (or shining curtain) occur in the choroid coating at the back of the eye, between the retina and the dark-colored sclera behind. The majority of hoofed mammals are equipped with a *fibrosum* type of choroid tapetum lucidum, wherein dense, regular strata of fibrous, sinewy connective tissues lie in glistening laminae. Nocturnal members of the primitive primate group and most carnivores of the cat family are equipped with a more complex structure, the *tapetum cellosum,* comprising wide, thin, and tilelike living endothelial cells of the kind present in choroid tissues. The numbers of such cells per layer of reflective elements (i.e., in cross section) range widely, from four or five in the wolverine to fifteen in the domestic cat, and up to thirty-five in some seals.

The light-reflecting tapeta are not situated in the choroid of all animals which exhibit nocturnal eyeshine. In some species *retinal tapeta* occur instead. Among such animals the best-known examples are found in deep-sea fishes and in crocodilians. Herein, the principal reflecting retinal material is a specular, white, nitrogenous ring compound of the purine class, *guanine* (App., 66b). It is encountered occasionally also in the choroid tapeta of some fishes, such as the sturgeon. Retinal tapeta rarely supplant the choroid type in mammals, save in some unusual instances, such as in the eyes of fruit bats and the common opossum, *Didelphis virginiana.* In such instances, however, the reflecting retinal particles are believed not to be guanine, which seems to be limited to cold-blooded animals.

Students of the subject suggest that an animal having a highly specular, reflective type of tapetum lucidum should thus gain in the ability to see and identify objects against their background under conditions of very faint light, thus facilitating the recognition of predators as well as prey.

Some further comments are called for about the white compound guanine, now with reference to its appearance in other body parts.

The integument of fishes offers various aspects of schemochromy. First, as to the striking, often glittering whiteness of the undersurface of much of the body (the so-called fish-belly-white feature): this is attributable to the presence of large numbers of epidermal *guanophores,* sometimes also called *iridocytes,* notably in the scales. These specialized cells are gorged with white, flakelike crystals of guanine, believed to be responsible also for the silvery appearance of some scales and the lateral lines in some species. The same compound is involved in the blueness of some fishes' skins, viewed at a vertical angle as well as the bright, specular blue patches adorning the body skin of juvenile "marine goldfish" or Garibaldi (*Hypsypops rubicunda*), whereas the bright orange-skinned adult of this species exhibits residual thin, blue stripes only along the fringes of fins and tail (pl. 13).

The thin, pigment-free platelets of guanine within some scales reflect interference-produced light fractions within restricted blue wavelengths, due to critical dimensions of thinness, while most of the incident light passes through, to be absorbed by layers of black melanin underlying the specular platelets.

Purely structural, schemochromic coloration seems to be very limited in the plant kingdom. No single instance of Tyndall-blue scattering comes to mind. Blueness of blossoms is derived from the presence of water-soluble pigments, as will be discussed briefly later.

There are, however, some instances of iridescence in plants. Among these are some seaweeds, as viewed when immersed. Some examples include red algae, such as *Iridophycus* spp., *Chondria californica, Cryptonemia obovata,* and *Schizymenia pacifica,* as well as the brown species *Zonaria farlowii.* The basis for spectral color expression in such plants seems not to have received detailed study. There are but few land plants exhibiting iridescence. Among these are to be found some of the *Lycopodium* mosses, and the upper surfaces of the pinnae or leaflets of a few true ferns, such as *Anemia makrinii. Selaginella* species, for example, *S. wildenovii* (pl. 3), native to damp forests in Malaysia, displays striking changeable blue coloration on the upper surfaces of its leaflets, whether in sunlight or shade. The chromatic effect is reminiscent of that in *Morpho* butterfly wings, but is less brilliant in the plant. The changeable colors in the plant are produced in the same basic manner as in the insect's wings, namely owing to countless very minute air spaces. The architecture differs in the two cases, however, for in *Selaginella* the chromatic features are called forth by the presence of countless microspheric, elevated air vesicles resembling masses of minute beadlets, highlighted on the upper, rounded, projecting surfaces, and manifesting successive blue, blue-green, purple, or violet hues according to the increasing angle of vision. When viewed at a maximal angle from the vertical—the so-called grazing angle—the optical colors vanish, leaving only the green color of chlorophyll.

The schemochromic colors of *Selaginella* disappear on wilting of the leaves. They are reversibly discharged on wetting the leaves briefly with water or alcohol, and they are restored on evaporation or blotting of the fluid. If, however, a true wetting agent of very low surface tension, such as in a detergent, be applied, the bright colors are quenched immediately and permanently as the beadlets of air are displaced from their adsorbed positions. Rinsing and blotting fails to restore the colors. In the intact plant, the tiny beadlets of air, inspected microscopically, are reminiscent of minute interstitial soap films and constitute the seat of color manifestation. The blue color seen from directly above is consistent with the bubblet films being thinnest at that locus.

OTHER SCHEMOCHROMIC SOURCES

To the three chief types of structurally colored entities, namely the whites of total scattered reflection, the Tyndall blues of selective scattering, and the iridescent features arising from interference between entering and returning light rays owing to multiple laminated surfaces, we should give at least passing attention to two others. These are (1) the spectral series evoked by prisms and certain other bodies through *refraction*, and (2) those resulting from *diffraction* of visible light, for example, by fine gratings. True, so-called prismatic refraction is seen most commonly in primary rainbows, resulting from the successive bending of sunlight components by myriads of spherical raindrops, affording to the viewer the familiar great spectral arcs across the sky.*

This particular manner of separation of light rays is rare, if known at all, in living organisms.

True diffraction, by natural gratings or very fine striae, resolves the incident light in a direct beam into its spectral components in an order opposite from the sequence in prismatic refraction, that is, involving maximal displacement of the longer (redward) and minimal of the shortest waves (see below). While of minor incidence in biological systems, diffraction iridescence has been reported in some species of the dark-brown, convex-bodied species of beetle in the genus *Serica*. Thus *S. sericea* shows no trace of iridescence when viewed only in diffused light, but if beams of light from a point source coincide with the line of vision *lengthwise* the curved elytra, two spectral orders are evident. Through an angle of 90°, colors appear in the bright, scintillating sequence: blue, green, yellow, orange, red; (purple), blue, green, orange, red. But if the line of vision and of light-beam impinge *crosswise* the elytra, no spectral colors are seen. The crosswise striae occur upon the very surface, each line being about 0.5 to 1 μ in depth, while interlinear spaces are very evenly about 0.8 μ in width, or some 30,000 per inch.

Sir Isaac Newton, in 1703, viewing on a screen the projected multiple color fringes diffracted by a single hair placed in the path of a narrow beam of sunlight, reported the increasing magnitude of diffraction of light rays in three orders: (1) violet, indigo, pale blue, green, yellow, red; (2) blue, yellow, red; and (3) pale blue, pale yellow, and red.

In the great majority of schemochromic manifestations by animals, whether in living tissues, such as skin or iris, or inanimate structures, including feathers or insect wings or elytra,

---

*"Monie a mickle mak's a muckle!" The murmured, contemplative words of Sandy (from Pitlochry, Perthshire), the handyman, looking skyward and summing up what he understood of the explained integrating refractive effects of billions of falling, spherical water drops, to give the huge, spectral arcs, primary and sometimes secondary or even additional orders.

underlying strata of dark pigment, usually melanin, are present. If the melanin layer is removed from a structure, whether by scraping with a sharp blade or, better, by oxidation with hydrogen peroxide, the original blue or multicolored object assumes a dull brown appearance, reminiscent of a dry leaf or a piece of brown paper. But if now the underside is painted with India ink, the schemochromic color is restored to the upper, reflecting surface, through the resumed absorption of all light-wave fractions which penetrate through the upper layers.

3
Carotenoids*

Any color, so long as it's red,
Is the color that suits me best,
Though I will allow there is much to be said
For yellow and green and the rest.
                                    Eugene Field

Whether on fruit, or lobsters or fish,
Or e'en on a lowly mould,
He is working, any of these are his dish;
But *I'll* gladly have emeralds and gold.
                                    L-G

In the green world of plants, enclosing and supporting the red kingdom of animals, no two classes of biochromes are more widely and continuously evident, nor of greater vital importance, than the porphyrins (App., 54-58) and the carotenoids (App., 1-30) not to mention being prime choices for pigments in the domain of the graphic arts. They are therefore subjects of greater scientific study.

Porphyrins are large, cyclic, complex, nitrogenous molecules (e.g., a-hematin, from hemoglobin, has a molecular weight of 633.32); they will be discussed in a later chapter. Suffice it to mention in passing the prominent inclusion of chlorophyll, the all-important green pigment of all photosynthetic plants; of hemoglobin, the oxygen-transporting chromoprotein in all red-blood animals; and of certain inconspicuous trace derivatives such as cytochrome, catalase, and other biocatalysts, or enzymes, which serve important biochemical functions in cellular metabolism.

*Pls. 10-33; App., 1-30.

Carotenoid molecules also are large, but linear, usually with cyclic structures at either terminal. They contain multiple double-bond loci, between alternate pairs of carbon atoms in the long, 18-carbon chain; hence they are so-called chemically unsaturated compounds involving carbon and hydrogen, and often also minor numbers of oxygen atoms, but no combined nitrogen.

A brief digression will outline the intramolecular features which are responsible for the evocation of colors as a result of the selective absorption of visible light fractions lying between the approximate wavelengths of 400 nm (violet) and 700 nm (deep red region). To repeat, light energy absorbed is converted into heat, while the residual, unabsorbed rays may then be observed through reflection or transmission. The capacity of a compound for absorbing visible light fractions arises from loci or special intramolecular nexuses called chromophores, or color-evoking configurations, within. These active sites are generated by chemically unsaturated bonding between neighboring atoms of carbon in the carotenoids (also between carbon and nitrogen atoms in porphyrins and bilichromes; see below); the double bonds created lead to a retardation in the vibrational frequency of the multiple electron pairs linking together neighboring atoms within a molecule. Sufficient modification in electronic vibrational frequency imparts to the whole molecule a special resultant or integrative motion—a chemical *resonance,* which, through internal friction, absorbs incident light rays of matching frequency, degrading that frequency to the level of heat waves; the remaining, unaffected light fraction is relayed to the observer's eye as a predominant color.

If a compound's molecular resonance corresponds to the frequency of short, rapid light waves, these become the fraction absorbed, that is, ones lying in the violet and blue regions; the emergent color is consequently yellow or orange. Compounds characterized by longer resonance frequencies neutralize incident light from the blue-green to green spectral regions, thus again affording colors in the orange to red realms. Finally, blue and green compounds acquire their colors from resonance cancellation of incident light in the long-waved orange or red end of the spectrum. Absorption of all incident light equally and completely gives a substance a black appearance, whereas white materials reflect equally and completely all light in the visible spectrum, absorbing only in the ultraviolet regions.

The color observed in a pigment usually includes some light from most of the visible spectrum except the absorbed fraction. The commonly observed color of a compound thus is dependent on the wavelength of the complementary, *dominant* fraction transmitted or reflected. The blue color of an aqueous copper sulfate solution, for example, is the result of a very broad band of light absorption showing a maximum, but not sole, effect in the red area of the spectrum.

The particular interatomic bonds which serve as chromophores or color-evoking entities within a molecule (with special reference here to the living world) are the chemically unsaturated linkages between alternate pairs of carbon atoms in a long chain, such as the 18-C chain in carotenoids; the similar double bonds in quinones or quinoid ring structures, supplemented by the presence of oxygenated carbon atoms at certain neighboring sites; and some carbon-to-nitrogen double-bonded ring configurations as well, occurring in the porphyrins and bilichromes (see App., 54-58, 60-64).

To return now to specific biochromes under discussion, let us first reflect upon the natural history of porphyrins and carotenoids, and perhaps touch on the subject of their presumptive evolutionary sequences.

In the first place, no animal synthesizes carotenoids *de novo;* the phenomenon occurs only in plant organisms, so far as is yet known. It involves not only all green plants, but many non-photosynthetic species as well, i.e., those found among the fungi and bacteria. Chlorophyll therefore appears not to be necessary for carotenoid synthesis. In fact, there are many instances of carotenoids occurring even in species which usually are green but which have grown in absence of all light; hence they are incapable of synthesizing chlorophyll, while exhibiting the yellow colors of the carotenoids. Furthermore, many fungal and bacterial species are able to synthesize carotenoids in completely dark environments. Moreover, rich supplies of the same compounds occur in some buried roots, such as in *Daucus carota,* the common carrot (whence, incidentally, this class of natural pigments received its name, dating from carotene's isolation by Wachenroder in 1826, some 150 years ago). There are, however, no instances of the occurrence of chlorophyll in the absence of carotenoids.

Animals obtain their carotenoids solely by devouring plants or plant remains, or by preying on other animal species which themselves may be herbivores or carotenoid-rich detritus feeders. Yet carotenoids serve vitally important functions in both plants and animals. Certain of these yellow or orange-colored compounds are responsible for many organisms' awareness of light, notably in the blue-to-green spectral regions, promoting their orientation, growth, or migration toward such light sources. Sighted animals utilize A vitamins, themselves colorless or faintly yellow carotenoid compounds whose presence in the retina of the eye implement the biochemical processes involved in vision. It is probable, indeed, that eyes and the pigments active in visual processes first evolved in animals living beneath the water's surface, where the most deeply penetrating visible fraction of sunlight displays a maximum intensity in the blue-green region, centering on about 568 nm in somewhat turbid waters near shorelines. Moreover, vitamin A plays an important role in growth and development and in implementing the integrity of animals' mucous surfaces. Its lack in the diet of humans and other vertebrates leads to drying of eye surfaces (xerophthalmia) and of the mouth and upper digestive tract (xerosis), thus permitting the occurrence of infection at such sites.

Certain porphyrins, for example, the cytochromes, in view of their indispensable role in cellular oxidation processes, may well be the most primitive biochromes of all. Yet the carotenoids could hardly have followed very far behind the early porphyrins in a relative sense; they probably even preceded the elaboration of chlorophyll itself. Heterotrophic organisms (feeders upon preformed organic molecules) assuredly had to come before the emergence of green, photosynthetic plants with their chlorophyll packets. yet carotenoid-synthesizing organisms might well have been present, some even needing the compounds for photosensitive orientation toward or away from vital, environmental light sources.

Pyrrole derivatives, fundamental to the ultimate structure of the vital tetrapyrroles (porphyrins and their kindred class, the bilichromes), are synthesized *de novo* by *both* plants and animals, which thus depend on no other source but themselves. The elaboration of chlorophyll, however, is restricted to the plant world, unless one cares to cite such instances as the interesting single-celled flagellate "phytozoan" (plant-animal) *Euglena,* which generates chlorophyll when living in lighted surroundings, thus enabling itself to live independently of an organic food supply. If transferred to a dark environment, however, it loses the green pigment and swallows microparticulate food, thus living as an animal.

While hemoglobins, on the other hand, are regarded as strictly characteristic of the animal kingdom (although not present in all animals), such hemoproteins are generated also in the root nodules of leguminous plants that harbor the symbiotic *Rhizobium* bacteria. Both the legume's nodule cells and the resident bacterial symbionts are required for the synthesis of this so-called leghemoglobin, which is not regarded here as an oxygen-transporting agent but as a biocatalyst serving an extraordinary role in the vitally important fixation of atmospheric nitrogen.

Passing reference has been directed to the prevailing colors of large bodies of water, and to the fact that the blue colors which characterize oceanic regions and some large lakes may be seasonally modified, or even replaced in limited areas, where one sees green from the blue-scattering, combined now with the yellow color of millions of single-celled plants—the phytoplankton; or other hues such as orange, red, or purple may arise from blooms of other single-celled plant or animal species. The so-called red tides, better named "red waters," provide common examples of such seasonally passing chromatic effects, which usually occur mostly in near-shore waters.

These yellow, orange, and red colors arise from the responsible cells' content of any of several representatives of the fat-soluble, carotenoid class of biochromes, formerly referred to by the old name of lipochromes, or by a modern chemical term polyenes (denoting their polyunsaturated character). The presence of these pigments in living things usually is measured only in milligrams or fractions thereof per 100 grams, or sometimes per kilogram, of tissue wet weight.

The marine phytoplankton constitute by far the world's most productive biochemical factory, synthesizing some 40 billion metric tons of organic matter by dry weight annually. A conservative estimate of but 0.01 percent of this quantity, say 10 mg/ 100 g, representing the carotenoid content of the product, still is equivalent to several hundred million tons of such compounds manufactured each year. The newly elaborated chlorophylls would exceed the carotenoid figure by severalfold. Chlorophylls, however, are even less stable chemically than are carotenoids and hence cannot be expected to persist unchanged for long.

There are two chief classes of carotenoids: (1) the carotenes (App., 1-5), which are highly unsaturated hydrocarbons, corresponding to an empirical formula of $C_{40}H_{56}$, of molecular weight 536.85; and (2) the xanthophylls (App., 6 et seq.) which are oxygenated carotenes, that is, with one or more hydroxyl (-OH) radicals or ketone ($=C=O$) groups substituted, usually at particular sites on the terminal rings. There are acidogenic xanthophyllic members also, which behave as, or can give rise to, acidic compounds. The Appendix provides a labeled list of the more common carotenoids directed toward the more interested reader.

Brown and yellow algal plants, saltwater and freshwater, synthesize, along with carotenes and greater quantities of xanthophylls, a predominant fraction, fucoxanthin, $C_{42}H_{58}O_6$ (App., 14). Various green terrestrial plants are likely to produce major proportions of the commoner, more conventional xanthophylls, such as lutein, zeaxanthin, and some others, but in some instances unusual members of the same class are encountered as well.

All are familiar with the yellow, orange, sometimes red colors of carotenoids in various blossoms and in fruits such as lemons, oranges, peaches, apricots, corn, melon flesh, tomatoes, and so on. Some ripe red berries, however, and the roots of radishes and beets owe their color to the presence of a different family of pigments, the water-soluble, acid-base-color-sensitive anthocyans, to be considered in a later chapter.

Carotenoid synthesis proceeds in many fruits during the

ripening stages, their colors often deepening with the passage of time. Replacement of chlorophyll in the skin of oranges and certain squashes by these yellow pigments is a familiar sight, as are the changes from green to yellow in pears and bananas stored after picking.

The color of carotenoid compounds deepens in proportion to the numbers of alternating double-bond pairs in the long chromophoric (chain) part of the molecule. Thus the carrot root, characterized by a preponderance of β-carotene, and containing nine double-bond pairs in the chain (App., 2) has a yellow-to-orange color, while γ-carotene, carrying ten such alternating or so-called conjugated pairs (App., 3) confers the deeper orange-to-red colors on marsh dodder, the parasitic threadlike plant that infests legumes and other green plants. Lycopene, the deep-red carotenoid responsible for the color of ripe tomatoes and the flesh of watermelons, bears eleven such double-bonded pairs (App., 5). We shall deal in greater detail with the carotenoids stored and metabolized by different animal phyla.

It may be useful to provide interested readers an abbreviated list of diagnostic features which characterize these pigments, as follows:

1. Color in living tissues or other parts: red, orange, yellow; in certain invertebrates blue, green, violet, brownish, gray or other combinations, due to conjugation with protein.

2. Solubility in various fat solvents: for example, alcohol, ether, benzene, chloroform, or hexane, following denaturation of tissue proteins.

3. Color in solution: yellow, orange, or red, depending on solvent, concentration therein, and chemical properties of the compound.

4. Color reaction with reagents: carotenoids dissolved in chloroform afford blue or green colors on mixing with concentrated sulfuric acid or with a chloroformic solution of antimony trichloride.

5. Partition test: pigment's distribution between hexane and 95 percent methanol:

    a) Carotenes and xanthophyllic *esters* of higher fatty acids remain *epiphasic,* that is, in upper layer of hexane.

    b) Free xanthophylls (whether naturally so or after hydrolsis) migrate down into the lower layer of 95 percent methanol, thus are *hypophasic*.

c) Certain acidogenic carotenoids, on treatment with alkali in presence of atmospheric oxygen, yield soaps which, on dilution of the system, now gather at the fluid interface.

6. Adsorptive chromatography: Separation of the different fractions into colored zones may be effected by passing a hexane solution of extract containing mixed carotenoids downward through packed columns in special glass tubes, or allowing the solvent to travel up across glass plates thinly layered with adsorbent powders, such as calcium carbonate (which adsorbs xanthophylls but not carotenes), or silica and magnesium oxide, or mixtures of these (which adsorb carotenes as well).

7. Spectroscopy: Dissolved in specified solvents, such as hexane, methanol, pyridine, or others, members of this pigment class give characteristic maximal absorption peaks, usually distributed within the blue, blue-green, and green regions, often with a minor peak in the violet range.

Being subject to degradation in the presence of light, atmospheric oxygen, elevated temperatures, or combinations of these, carotenoids should be stored, awaiting analysis, in glass-stoppered vessels containing a nitrogen atmosphere, within a dark, cold space such as a refrigerator.

Carotenoids ingested with food by animals are subject to any of several alternative, but not necessarily mutually exclusive, fates, as follows:

1. Rejection via feces, in chemically unchanged condition.

2. Assimilation and storage in an unmodified state.

3. Assimilation and conversion into another carotenoid, usually by adding or substituting oxygen atoms into the molecule— for example, β-carotene ($C_{40}H_{56}$, App., 2) may be converted to astaxanthin ($C_{40}H_{52}O_4$, App., 22), and β-carotene may also be split and oxidized to give two molecules of vitamin A (retinal), of empirical formula $C_{20}H_{28}O$ (App., 30).

4. Assimilated portions completely oxidized.

Actually, several of these processes occur in an animal organism: some is wasted, some oxidatively consumed, and some stored, either unchanged or modified. However, the conversion of one carotenoid into another colored, nonvitamin member is specific for certain animals, as we shall observe below.

Animals which consume and deal metabolically with carotenoids have been grouped into the following five general types, typifying the above principal alternative dispositions:

1. "Carotene" animals assimilate specifically, and store only, or chiefly, the hydrocarbon type, or carotenes (horse, cow, some invertebrates).

2. "Xanthophyll" animals selectively assimilate and store only the alcoholic and hydroxylated, xanthophyllic members, and perhaps some ketonic types as well in some instances, rejecting the carotenes in the feces or degrading them through metabolic oxidation; they convert some of the carotene into A vitamins (domestic fowl and other birds, most fishes, many invertebrates).

3. Nonselective animals readily assimilate and store both hydrocarbon and oxygenated classes of carotenoid (man, frog, octopus).

4. "Noncarotenoid" animals store very few or no carotenoids of either class, whether through complete voidance in feces or oxidative degradation in the body, although, like the rest, they can oxidatively split carotene to yield vitamin A (swine, Carnivora, sheep, goats, and a few invertebrates).

5. Carotenoid innovators assimilate various carotenoids and convert them by oxidation into derivatives, usually of increased molecular weight, e.g., β-carotene ($C_{40}H_{56}$) $\rightarrow$ zeaxanthin ($C_{40}H_{56}O_2$, App., 8) $\rightarrow$ canthaxanthin ($C_{40}H_{52}O_2$, App., 20) $\rightarrow$ astaxanthin ($C_{40}H_{50}O_4$, App., 22) (crustaceans, some fishes, certain birds, including flamingo, scarlet ibis, roseate spoonbill).

It hardly needs to be reemphasized that the respective metabolic dispositions of ingested carotenoids are not mutually exclusive. All consumers, for example, are wasteful in that they reject some of the ingested compounds in their feces, and all consumers oxidatively destroy, in gut or tissues, a portion of the total supply. Moreover, whereas selectivity of a certain class of carotenoid may be dependent on an animal's predominant disposition of the available supply, this is not to say that there may not be minor amounts of the other class assimilated and in some instances even stored. Finally, we have observed that all animals, or certainly all vertebrates and perhaps many invertebrates, are capable of the oxidative splitting of carotene to yield vitamin A aldehyde, often called retinal from its presence and role in the retina; its molecular weight amounts to somewhat more than half that of the parent carotene: β-carotene ($C_{40}H_{56}$: m.w. = 536.85) + O_2 $\longrightarrow$ 2 retinals ($C_{20}H_{28}O$: m.w. = 284.44). The increase in molecular weight contributed by 2 atoms of oxygen, yielding theoretically 2 molecules of retinal, is a total of 32.

With this brief introductory outline for reference, supplemented optionally by consultation of the Appendix for structural formulas of the various carotenoids, we may now consider a few representative animals from among the more prominent phyla. More inclusive and detailed coverage is to be found in *Animal Biochromes* and other works listed in the Bibliography.

PROTOZOA
(single-celled animals)

It is important to recall that, under this heading, there may be some confusion between certain flagellated unicellular animal forms and a few members of flagellated unicellular plant species, to which we have referred, for convenience, as *phytozoa,* or plant-animals. All chlorophyll-bearing flagellates are naturally to be classed as plant species, in view of their capacity for photosynthesis, lacked by true animals. It has been observed, however, that certain single-celled species, such as *Euglena gracilis,* exhibit both plant and animal characteristics. These green euglenoid flagellates, manufacturing their own food through photosynthesis, lose their chlorophyll when cultured in darkness, and become not only saprophytic, utilizing soluble organic matter as do bacteria and fungi, but turn into animalcules as well, in that they engulf finely particulate food via the cytostome or mouth-organelle. The carotenoids remain most concentrated in the conspicuous red stigma, or so-called eyespot, situated near the forward, flagellated end of the elongate body.

Some protophytes, including certain phytozoan species, are encountered within the tissues of protozoan and other invertebrate hosts, often conferring upon such commensal partners a considerable degree of coloration. Varying degrees of unilateral or mutual metabolic dependence exist between the resident plant organisms and their animal hosts.

A number of protozoans, notably radiolarians, as well as Porifera (sponges), Coelenterata (among which are the anemones, corals, and jellyfish or siphonophores), as well as a few worm species, marine snails, and bivalved molluscs including the tridachnids or giant clams, colonial ascidians (sea-squirts), some bryozoa (moss-animals), and echinoderms belong to the host group harboring single-celled plant colonies. Such resident plants doubtless profit from assimilating some of the soluble organic wastes of the host animal, which in turn acquires direct transfer of oxygen, and perhaps soluble nutrients as well, for its tissues.

Anemones such as *Anthopleura xanthogrammica,* the common, large, usually green species prolific along the shores of the North American Pacific Coast, is a conspicuous example of an animal host, bearing within its tissues colonies of unicellular algae or zooxanthellae in a symbiotic or mutually beneficial relationship. Green-colored due to the presence of chlorophyll in the algal cells, in well-lighted zones, these anemones are white, or of their own pinkish or pale lavender colors under subdued illumination, when they carry no algal symbionts.

Yellow, orange, or ruddy coloration observed in snow and in rain ponds and other freshwater bodies, sea patches and saline waters, or naturally concentrated brines (pl. 26) owe their identity to the presence of myriads of free-living unicellular algae.

Chalmydomonas nivalis is characteristic of "red snow" and "red rain" in puddles, ditches, and bog ponds, which also afford rich populations of such algal cells as *Haematococcus pluvialis;* whereas marine areas of "red water" are evoked by blooms of the dinoflagellate *Gonyaulax polyedra,* reaching populations of several million cells per liter in Southern California waters. Similar eruptions of another dinoflagellate, *Proro-*

centrum micans, can give rise to yellowish or orange colors, while other forms contribute dirty brown or chocolate-colored aspects. All such manifestations arise from the presence of rich concentrations of carotenoids within the cells.

Dunaliella salina, a red, biflagellated algal species which characterizes the red colors of concentrated, natural brines, owes the coloration to its storage of substantial amounts of β-carotene (pl. 26). The colors of such brines are particularly rich in summer and fall, notably in temperate sites such as prevail in California. Earlier in the year, before evaporation has proceeded so far, the saline waters are green, not only due to *D. salina's* own greenness with much chlorophyll in springtime, but also from the presence of an allied, smaller biflagellate species, *D. viridis,* which gradually is replaced by increasingly greater populations of *D. salina* as the salts become more concentrated. Some students of the species believe that the two forms are conspecific, that is, of the same species, but variable in size, shape, and predominant color owing to external factors of salinity and perhaps temperature.

Referring again to plant cells living within animal hosts' tissues, such floral adornments not only fortuitously augment the beauty of their cultivating carriers, but may, more often than not, provide distinct economic advantages. Consider, for example, *Velella lata* (pl. 30), the beautiful little blue siphonophore, a colonial coelenterate equipped with a rigid sail, permanently erected at a slightly diagonal angle across the long axis of the ovate, somewhat flattened mantle. *Velella* carries within its endodermal tissues a gorged mass of tiny, rounded, brownish-yellow, carotenoid-rich algal cells,* or zooxanthellae, seen collectively as an extensive brown area in the middle part of the dorso-ventrally flattened, oval-shaped body.

The relationship between the coelenterate host, *Velella,* and its algal plants actually is symbiotic, that is, mutually beneficial, rather than being merely commensal. Since *Velella* floats con-

---

*These appear golden yellow individually under magnification. The brown color of their appearance en masse, in situ, arises from the combined carotenoid-yellow and chlorophyll-green. Zooxanthellae commensal in other species may exhibit lighter or heavier shades of brownish hue depending on the ratios of the two classes of pigment present.

tinually on the sea surface, it exposes the crop of algal flora to ample daily sunlight, filtered, however, through the blue "window" of its mantle, thus precluding solarization, or overexposure, yet transmitting ample light to permit photosynthesis within the algal cells.

The symbiotic algae, thus afforded safe carriage, ample continuous and controlled light quanta, and provided with certain soluble, nutritious compounds through the host's metabolic wastes, doubtless repay their manager not only with minor amounts of freshly manufactured glucose but demonstrably with ample photosynthetically evolved oxygen gas, which diffuses into the animal's multiple air canals, situated between the endoderm, bearing the plant cells, and the upper mantle surface. This surplus oxygen supply ensures the animal colony's ability to remain afloat, upper surface exposed. Therefore it not only is removed from maximum exposure to attack from predacious animals, but functions in an optimal locus for encountering food in the form of small planktonic animals and plant eggs, as well as organic remains or other detritus. All of these tend to float, being of lower specific gravity than seawater, and thus can be sensed and seized by the colony's tentacles.

There are some true Protozoa that are richly colored red, orange, or yellow, in all probability by carotenoids. A seasonally red species, *Euglena sanguinea,* reportedly exhibits its maximal coloration in spring and autumn, in bright sunshine, when surrounding conditions are somewhat dry. This species, however, is a phytozoan. Of true protozoans displaying carotenoid pigmentation we learn of shell-forming animals, including *Globigerina* species, which aggregate to give floating, scarlet-hued blooms atop the ocean surface. Among other foraminifera, *Myxotheca arenilega* is a relatively large single-celled type whose whole protoplast is tinted by a fine-grained Pompeian red pigment, perhaps derived from brightly colored microcrustaceans devoured by the protozoan.

Violet, rose, green, or blue pigments occur in certain infusorian (ciliated) protozoans. A species of *Spirophyra* digests the colored eye material of the copepod *Idya furcata,* thus robbing it of its carotenoid pigment. Species of *Polyspira* and *Gymnodinioides* similarly parasitize the hermit crab *Eupagurus pridauxii,* depriving it of its ocular pigment. In such instances, the small, parasitic protozoan digests with the food vacuole the blue carotenoid protein of its host's eye. The red carotenoid residue is then assimilated and recombined with a new protein, adorning the parasitic infusorian with resulting violet, blue, or other colors. During reproductive division, or fission of the cells, the acquired pigment is partitioned among the newly generated daughter cells.

PORIFERA
(sponges)

The sponges are sedentary, comparatively simple, colonial animal forms, occurring in various shapes and sizes and often with pronounced variations in pigmentation. Many display gray or other drab, inconspicuous aspects, while numerous species are colored brilliantly red, orange, yellow, purple, or actually black. The brighter pigments of sponges have prompted published studies by biologists for nearly a century; doubtless they have been the subject of abiding interest for far longer.

A number of species bearing carotenoids are mentioned in *Animal Biochromes* (1976). The discussion is notable for its inclusion of references to somewhat older works, wherein little information is found as to carotenoid identities in the species in question.

The red sponge *Axinella crista-galli* contains the red, acidogenic carotenoid astaxanthin, and another red carotenoid reportedly occurs in yet another sponge, *Suberites domuncula,* which is believed to store the red hydrocarbon torulene, typical in the red yeast *Torula rubra;* α-, β-, and γ-carotenes also were suspected in the same sponge, as well as in another, *Ficulina ficus.*

The red sponge *Hymeniacidon sanguineum* has been found to yield both echinenone, the orange-colored monoketonic provitamin A compound common in sea urchins, and γ-carotene, the deepest colored member of the carotene series (see App., 19a, 3).

Most unusual of the sponge carotenoids are the rare aromatic compounds, that is, those carrying trimethylbenzene rather than trimethylcyclohexenyl rings, one at either end of the chain. Outstanding members of this class are renieratene, isoreniera-tene, and renieropurpurin, isomeric compounds differing one from another only in the relative positions of the methyl radicals attached to the terminal benzoid rings, and in the spatial relationship of these to the points of attachment of the rings to the central chain (see App., 27, 28, and 29).

V. Elliott Smith has done some of the most recent critical analytical work on sponge carotenoids. He studied the histological and biochemical features of two red poriferan species in particular, namely *Trikentrion helium* and *Cyamon neon,* both in the family Cyamonidae, and occurring in the same bottom environment beneath the coastal waters off Southern and Baja California.

The two species are strikingly similar as to pigmentary composition, but differ widely in disposition of carotenoids in so-called chromatocytes. In chromatocytes of *T. helium* it seems that relatively polar lipids or fatlike substances bind chemically with protein and carry carotenoids in a water-soluble condition. Contrasting with this, pigmented granules occur within the chromatocytes of *C. neon* wherein a specific protein carrier, and perhaps bonded lipids as well, seem to be lacking. In this species the xanthophylls are largely esterified, which fact, rendering them less polar, should also impart mutual solubility with the lipids, and perhaps greater chemical stability as intracellular granules.

Chemical and spectrophotometric analyses of chromatographically separated fractions revealed ten or eleven different compounds in each of the two species. The respective fractions were surprisingly similar qualitatively, though differing quantitatively in certain instances. The yields amounted to 42.4 and 43.4 percent of the fractions as hydrocarbons of rare type, for *Trikentrion* and *Cyamon* respectively, while the remaining fractions were suspected to be largely monohydroxy with a few ketonic carotenoids.

These sponges thus are consistent with earlier observed features involving relatively high proportions of the hydrocarbon type of stored carotenoid. Moreover, the kinds of compound encountered were rare. No evidence was found to suggest whether these sponges acquire their bizarre carotenoid fractions through introducing innovations into more conventional carotenoids ingested, or whether, as would seem more probable, they gain the unusual fractions directly through consumption of microorganisms that may manufacture and store such pigments.

Certainly, in their storage of relatively high proportions of the hydrocarbon or monohydroxy hydrocarbon types of carotenoid, as well as in the comparative rarity of such types, the sponges are conspicuously in contrast to the great majority of invertebrate animal forms.

Smith appended to his dissertation a summarizing quotation from Gerard (1636), as follows:

"There is found, growing upon the rocks neer unto the sea a certaine matter wrought togither, of the forme or froth of the sea, which we call spunges...whereof to write at large woulde greatly increase our volume, and little profite the Reader."

COELENTERATA
(anemones, corals, hydroids, jellyfish)

The coelenterate phylum of animals assuredly is a rival for exhibition of the greatest variety and vividness of biochromy. The rich concentrations of colored compounds, mainly carotenoids, in their thin and watery tissues lend compelling emphasis to important questions surrounding the origin and significance of biochromes. *British Sea Anemones* (1928/1935) by the late T. A. Stephenson presents beautifully colored illustrations of many such species. Mention has been made concerning the blue colors of certain medusae or jellyfish; while some such pigments belong to a heterogeneous group of incompletely known chemical nature, a number of them have been established as conjugated carotenoid-proteins. *Velella* and *Porpita* are two examples of such blue forms; the blue chromoprotein in *Velella lata* (pl. 30) involves the oxygenated, acidogenic carotenoid astaxanthin, common among Crustacea and many other phyla. When the blue protein material is coagulated by heating or treatment with alcohol, or is denatured with acids or alkalis, the blue color disappears, giving place to the orange or red of the now liberated astaxanthin.

Current evidence points to the distribution of red, orange, yellow or other colored carotenoids, whether free or conjugated with protein, throughout nearly every branch of the coelenterate phylum. This is not to say that every species within the group carries colored carotenoids, for some of them are white, showing no pigmentation until egg-ripening season, when red or other characteristic colors may be seen through the body wall.

Nor are members of the carotenoid class confined to only the soft parts, for we have discovered several instances wherein polar (oxygenated) carotenoids, notably astaxanthin, are firmly bonded in some way with the calcareous skeleton in some hydrocoral species and in at least one of the gorgonians, or horny corals, often called sea fans. Again, none save relatively few coral species with brightly colored skeletons owe their bright appearance to the presence of carotenoids.

Of the few studied, mention should be made of the purple hydrocoral of Southern California waters, *Allopora californica* (pl. 31) which owes its permanent color (discharged only by heat or by dissolution of the calcareous material in acids) to the presence of astaxanthin, chemically bonded to protein as a bluish complex, and apparently linked also with the calcium. (Rønneberg et al., 1978).

A vermilion-colored skeleton from *Distichopora violacea,* a pink-and-red one from *D. coccinea,* and even a pale orange one from *D. nitida,* all yielded astaxanthin as the only carotenoid recoverable. Three species of *Stylaster* were investigated as well, and *S. rosea's* skeleton was found to contain astaxanthin as the sole carotenoid, while in the pink-and-orange skeleton of *S. elegans* and in the pale pink one from *S. sanguineus* the astaxanthin was accompanied by minor proportions of a neutral, suspectedly dihydroxy xanthophyll, also firmly bonded.

It is to be hoped that additional research will throw more light on the kinds of pigments investing colored coral skeletons, and concerning also the exact manner whereby polar carotenoid-proteins may be bonded to the carbonaceous skeleton.

The carotenoid pigmentation characterizing the many fleshy parts of coelenterates in general is, of course, far more brilliant and patterned than that responsible for the skeletal coloration of corals.

The anemone *Actinia equina* occurs in red, brown, and green varieties. The red form carries a red, ectodermal carotenoid, and the brown and green variants exhibit an orange one plus a green pigment dispersed in endodermal tissues. Specimens denied food, or raised from the egg stage upon carotenoid-free food, lack pigmentation; yet when allowed a carotenoid-rich diet of shrimp eggs, they assume their characteristic colors. The previously starved animals were found to be consistent in their resumption of original pigmentation: the originally red animals recovered their red color; the green and the brown forms resumed storage of their respective, earlier pigments. One red carotenoid fraction is unique, namely actinioerythrin, an oxygenated, acidogenic compound which occurs as an ester, and which is very unstable following hydrolysis. There occurs also a red-orange xanthophyll which, when conjugated with a protein by the animal, displays the green color. Violerythrin, another fraction discovered in the same anemone species, is also acidogenic, like astaxanthin and actinioerythrin (App., 24).

Unlike *Actinia, Anemonia sulcata* bears commensal algae which yield chlorophyll, carotenes, and peridinin, a xanthophyll typical of the plant cells. The similar storage of algal zooxanthelae in the tissues of *Anthopleura xanthogrammica* already has been mentioned.

Of the large numbers of brightly colored anemone species, few are more spectacular than the color variants of the widely occurring plumose anemone *Metridium,* with its feathery tentacles and greatly extensible column. Subspecies of the British and European form *M. senile* occur on the Atlantic and Pacific coasts of North America, namely *M. s. marginatum* and *M. s. fimbriatum* (pl. 27) respectively. This genus harbors no commensal algal cells, but exhibits a diversity of coloration in its tissues. There are all-white (the most commonly occurring variant), simple red, simple brown, and simple gray forms; moreover, there are various other genotypes that arise from crossing, such as red-with-brown, brown-with-gray, red-with-brown-with-gray, and others wherein there are white parts with red or brown. In such hybrids the variation among the colors is distributed between the outer surface of the body wall, the capitulum and tentacles, and the stomodaeum or mouth. There occur also rare orange or yellow-orange specimens. The carotenoids responsible for pigmentation, for example, in the red variant, occur in fat droplets in the base of ectodermal cells and are distributed throughout the endodermal cells lining the gastro-vascular cavity and coelenteron. Brown or gray genotypes have melanin, either diffuse or in fine, black aggregates (in the gray), instead of ectodermally stored carotenoids, while the endoderm remains colorless.

In the white phase, males remain pure matte white throughout the year, whereas females, retaining their all-white somatic tissues, seasonally develop pink to red eggs which remain in the then similarly colored ovarian tissues lining the free edges of the longitudinal septa within the enteron. This factor gives the female animal a soft pink appearance, notably when the column is expanded and viewed with adequate light.

Professor Carl Pantin and I, working at Cambridge University, discovered in color variants of *M. s. senile* the following general pigmentary qualities and compounds.

Color	Melanins	Carotenoids
White	None	Astaxanthin and *esters* thereof in ripe females.
Brown (various shades)	Varying degrees	Few; esters of astaxanthin and/or metridioxanthin; minor carotenes.
Yellow-orange	Little or none	Considerable; *metridioxanthin esters,* xanthophyll esters, carotenes, free xanthophylls.
Red with brown	Varying degrees	Many; esters of *metridioxanthin* and of *astaxanthin.*
Red	None	Many; *metridioxanthin esters,* sometimes with free or esterified astaxanthin; free metridioxanthin, carotenes, xanthophylls.

In the foregoing list the predominant carotenoid fractions are italicized. Any carotenes and common xanthophylls occurred in minor amounts.

At a later time, the study was resumed, with the assistance of G. F. Crozier and V. E. Smith, using the Pacific Coast subspecies, *M. s. fimbriatum,* with some comparative analyses of red *M. s. senile* variants from Britain.

Our Pacific *Metridium,* as well as those from Britain, yielded esterified astaxanthin esters as the principal carotenoid fraction recoverable from either somatic or ovarian tissues. Esters of a zeaxanthinlike xanthophyll often were found, notably in somatic tissues of the colored forms, while comparable parts in the white forms of both sexes were without pigment. In this series of analyses, no carotenes were detected in either the Pacific or the red British specimens. Astaxanthin always was dominant, and mostly in esterified form.

In more recent studies at La Jolla, D. W. Wilkie and I have searched for carotenoid precursors to astaxanthin in the natural diet of *Metridium* (pl. 27), which the anemone stores in esterified form in the ripe eggs. This red compound has been greatly predominant, often the only carotenoid found in the ova of the several colored genotypes studied (i.e, white, red, tan, brown, red-brown).

Large adult white females, segregated in aquariums with running seawater chilled to temperatures between 9° and 12°C, and hence simulating conditions in their natural habitat, received chowdered white fish muscle, supplemented with a particular carotenoid in each experimental series. From time to time ova were taken by syringe, through a hollow needle from the animal's enteron, and analyzed.

When fed a supplement of β-carotene as the sole carotenoid, the animals, although absorbing the pigment in their digestive tubules, failed completely to assimilate it into the developing ova or any body parts. Indeed, the development of colorless ova was discovered in *Metridium,* following a protracted period on the carotene-supplemented diet.

The same findings resulted when a dihydroxy-β-carotene derivative, zeaxanthin (App., 8) had been similarly administered. In this instance the animals stored little if any of the pigment even in the digestive tubules, nor any in the ova, which developed without color.

A successful carotenoid proved to be astaxanthin itself (App., 22), as administered in finely shredded red salmon flesh. The free pigment was esterified by the consumers and stored thus in the ripening ova.

Canthaxanthin (diketo-β-carotene, App., 20) was the only other, of many carotenoids tried, observed to be converted by *Metridium* into astaxanthin, which was esterified and stored in the ripening ova.

ECHINODERMATA
(sea stars, brittle stars, sea urchins, sea cucumbers)

In this, the echinoderm (literally spiny-skinned) phylum, we encounter a wide variety of forms, food and feeding habits, and coloration. Moreover, among the sea stars in particular, we find a great assortment of bright skin pigmentation, rivaling that of sea anemones. Animals in the asteroid class are carnivorous for the major part, subsisting upon living prey, as do the sea anemones, and yet storing the richest supplies of carotenoids. No such sweeping statement should be allowed to stand without citing one or two of the rare exceptions. Among the sea anemones, reviewed in the preceding section, it was found that *Metridium* is in fact an omnivore, subsisting on small planktonic plant and animal organisms and other fine particles; in the asteroid echinoderms there is the small, pointed sea star *Henricia,* which also consumes such small animals, plants, and organic residues, whether directly from the surrounding water or, more commonly, from submerged rock surfaces, where the crawling, exploring creature finds such food.

Asteroids (sea stars)

Representative analytical surveys have shown that the bright integument, as well as the pyloric caeca or digestive apparatus, in species of sea stars yield no more than traces of carotenes

proper, but commonly more than 90 percent of the total as xanthophyllic pigments, including substantial proportions of the
acidogenic pigment astaxanthin. Such species thus examined
have included the sand star *Astropecten californicus,* many colored phases of the webbed star *Patiria miniata* (pl. 20), and the
two large, very common and voracious predators found on
tidally exposed pier pilings and rocks, *Pisaster ochraceus,* the
ocher star which varies in skin color from yellow through
orange, purple, and brown and *P. giganteus,* the purple specimen. Both skin and pyloric caeca in all four species are rich in
carotenoids, and yield astaxanthin, or mytiloxanthin, an allied
acidogenic carotenoid found in *P. ochraceus,* which preys
heavily on the mussels *Mytilus californianus* and *M. edulis,*
wherein the same carotenoid has been identified. Astaxanthin
or a close chemical relative thereof is present also in the red- or
orange-tipped spines on the back of the soft star *Astrometis
sertulifera* (pl. 21).

The webbed star *Patiria miniata's* genotypic color variants of
yellow, orange, red, brown, or purple hue, or bearing certain
variegated color patterns, have been characterized in part by the
relative proportions of astaxanthin among the carotenoid fractions recoverable from the integument. Thus the respective
orange-, red-, brown-, and purple-skinned types yielded major
proportions of astaxanthin as follows: 51:40, 66:25, 72:21, and
80:19. The lesser fraction in each case is preponderantly neutral
xanthophyllic material, save for ca. 0.05 percent carotenes.

T. S. Hopkins has carried out an extensive investigation of
the carotenoids responsible for skin color in three species of the
small, pointed-rayed sea star *Henricia,* encountered in shallow
coastal waters of Southern California. The three forms studied
were *H. annectens* (Orange Chrome to Morocco Red), *H.
leviuscula* (Apricot Orange to Garnet Brown), and *H. palespina*
(Cadmium Yellow to Deep Vinaceous Rufous), a species described and named by Hopkins. The color designations were
taken from Ridgeway's 1912 standards.

Species within this genus vary in respect to most other sea
stars in two conspicuous ways. First, regarding their diet, as
observed, they are not predatory carnivores as are most asteroid

genera, but subsist upon leptopel or finely particulate suspended and settling detrital matter, as well as on microplank-
tonic animals and plants. Moreover, perhaps correlated with
the food habit is *Henricia*'s storage of the great preponderance
of its skin carotenoids as neutral oxygenated xanthophylls, the
carotenes amounting to less than 6 percent of the totals. These
findings are in line with the great predominance of xanthophylls
over carotenes in the living and detrital components of *Henricia*'s food. In this genus, however, astaxanthin itself is not a
prominent fraction of the xanthophylls stored, although certain
other ketonic carotenoids, related to astaxanthin, occur in
minor proportions.

An arresting instance of sexual dichromatism emerged among
these sea stars, in that males of *H. leviuscula* exhibited generally
darker skin colors than females, rendering it feasible to distin-
guish the sexes solely by this characteristic. The emergence of a
chromatic secondary sexual character in a benthic, sightless
invertebrate is indeed singular.

Another observation involved an orange-chrome male of *H.
palespina,* whose skin was without any of the acidogenic carotenoid material stored by females. An hermaphroditic specimen
(the only one encountered) of the same species stored prominently a β-carotenoic acid fraction normally encountered in but
minor proportions in animals of any of the three species.

Regeneration of pigmented epidermal skin was demonstrated
by scrubbing away the integument from two rays of an *H. palespina* specimen, and then enclosing it within an undersea cage
on a rocky floor for nearly 7 months before reanalyzing. Two
of the normal arms, serving as controls, yielded 31.43 mg carotenoids per 100 g of fresh original integument, while the fresh,
regenerated skin on the experimental arms, now fairly well colored but lighter, afforded a recovery of two-thirds of its pigment: 20 mg per 100 g. Moreover, the regenerated and control
skin samples yielded the same four carotenoid fractions.

Brightly pigmented patches, or so-called eye spots, one at the
tip of each ray, are believed by some investigators to serve as
light-sensitive organs, leading to movement by the animal,
whether toward or away from a source of illumination. *Martha-*

sterias glacialis carries yellowish-orange and reddish-orange loci in the optic cushion of each eye spot. β-Carotene and astaxanthin have been identified in the site.

Astropecten californicus, the rapidly moving sand star, possesses a purplish eye spot at the tip of each arm involving an astaxanthin chromoprotein. Its tube feet are unusual, being without adhesive or sucking pads; it gains its food at or beneath the surface of sandy floors and is responsive to light.

Ophiuroids (serpent stars or brittle stars)

Many animals in this echinoderm class exhibit, like asteroids, numerous bright colors, including blue, green, red, and yellow, characteristic of shallow-water members, and more often bright orange or red in abyssal forms. Even the numerous species of dull brownish, gray, or black aspect seem to be internally rich in carotenoids.

There have not been many analytical studies of ophiuran carotenoids, but B. T. Scheer and I studied three species in detail. Of the three, *Ophiopteris papillosa,* a dark gray to blackish brittle star, and two smaller and brilliantly colored species, *Ophiothrix spiculata* and *O. rudis,* none yielded any detectable carotenes; the epiphasic fractions (preferentially soluble in hexane over slightly aqueous methanol, as are all carotenes) all were esters of hydroxylated xanthophylls. Of these, several recoverable fractions included two new acidogenic carotenoids in each of the two *Ophiothrix* species; in the same two, the other ester involved a yellow xanthophyll showing an absorption spectrum reminiscent of taraxanthin or dinoxanthin. In another case, *O. papillosa* yielded about six-fold more free than esterified xanthophylls, again suspectedly dinoxanthin, typical of marine dinoflagellates.

The multiple fractions included several unique carotenoids, in some instances too chemically unstable to preserve for analysis or to survive it.

The few ophiuran species studied suggest that these animals are selective xanthophyll acceptors, rejecting carotenes, and that they may oxidize a portion of the assimilated xanthophylls to give unstable acidic or other more oxygenated products.

Echinoids (sand dollars, sea urchins)

Members of this class of echinoderms are noted for their storage, in skeleton and internal tissues, of rich deposits of polyhydroxynaphthoquinone (or echinochrome) pigments, to be discussed in a later chapter. Carotenoids are stored internally, notably in the gonadal tissues and in the gut, while any integumentary carotenoids are masked, either by dark melanins or by the above-mentioned red, purple, or greenish echinochromes.

The orange-colored gonadal mass (a food delicacy) of the urchin *Strongylocentrotus lividus* reportedly contains a- and β-carotenes in similar proportions, as well as approximately the same quantity of echinenone, a monoketone of β-carotene which, like the latter, is a provitamin A. There are larger proportions of xanthophylls, including some unusual, heavily oxygenated members, such as pentaxanthin (= isofucoxanthinol), derived from seaweeds consumed by the urchin.

The purple sand dollar *Dendraster excentricus* (pl. 8) and three sea urchin species, the red *Strongylocentrotus franciscanus* (pl. 7), the purple *S. purpuratus* (pl. 6), and *Lytechinus pictus,* a pale form, were examined for recoverable carotenoids.

All four species yielded β-carotene; *Lytechinus* and *S. purpuratus* contained a-carotene as well. The three urchins, and suspectedly the sand dollar too, carried echinenone. There were xanthophylls resembling zeaxanthin or diatoxanthin (which have similar absorption spectra), lutein or pentaxanthin, and a few then lesser-known members such as peridinin. The xanthophylls were, for the most part, uncombined as esters, appearing only partly esterified, and variably, in *S. purpuratus.*

Male *Dendraster* specimens excelled females in carotenoid content, rating twice the concentration of β-carotene plus echinenone and thrice the quantity of xanthophylls retrieved from females. The endoderm yielded only traces of either class of carotenoid, while the intestine was richest and the gonads high in second place.

In the purple urchin, intestinal levels of both carotenes and xanthophylls are relatively high, about equally so in both sexes, xanthophylls preponderating by about twofold. However, ovarian exceeded spermary tissues in carotene content by about threefold; and in neither sex were any gonadal xanthophylls found. In *Lytechinus,* relatively high levels of carotenes and echinenone are stored in the gonads, the testicular material being particularly high in them, while xanthophylls occur also, in secondary concentrations, in both ovaries and spermaries.

Females of the purple urchin and of *Lytechinus* carry about one-fourth of their total carotenoids in the ovaries, whereas the respective males mobilize one-sixth and one-third to the spermaries although the sperm itself is, of course, uncolored. Beyond doubt the ovarian carotenoid content may be expected to vary seasonally as the eggs ripen and later as they are discharged.

Holothurians (sea cucumbers)

Representatives of this class, like the others, frequently are found to have carotenoids in the digestive gland and particularly in the ovaries. Such species as *Mesothuria intestinalis* bear yellow or red (ripe) ovaries, while some specimens of *Cucumaria lactea* and *Ocnius brunneus* have blue-to-pale-blue ovaries, due to the presence of a red carotenoid, probably astaxanthin, conjugated with protein. Several other holothurian species display carotenoid pigmentation in their gonads, while having whole bodies of an externally yellow-brown color. *Stichopus parvimensis,* a common brown cucumber in coastal waters of Southern California, yields very small, equal amounts of carotenes and xanthophylls from its body skin.

Another species, *Cucumaria lubrica,* carries a high content of free astaxanthin in its red body wall.

Crinoids (sea lilies)

These animals, whether attached to rocks on the sea floor or as free-swimming forms, may exhibit brown, red, purple, violet, green, yellow, or even black coloration; yet little indeed has been learned of any carotenoids assimilated and stored by them. The free-swimming form *Antedon* does yield carotenoids in minor amounts, but here, as with the majority of colored crinoids, pigments other than carotenoids are responsible, as we shall see later.

If one accepts the division of the echinoderm phylum into two chief feeding groups, namely carnivores, including the asteroids and ophiuroids, and the echinoids and holothurians, which subsist principally on detritus and on certain plant materials (but are to some extent omnivores), one encounters some interesting quantitative correlations as to carotenoid metabolism in the respective types. Carnivorous species seem to store three- to fourfold the quantities of such pigments found in the herbivore-detritophagous species. Moreover, the bulk of carotenoids found in the carnivores belong to the heavily oxygenated compounds, including notable carotenoid acids or acidogenic members, which are rare or lacking in the other group.

MOLLUSCA
(bivalves, snails or slugs, cephalopods)

Again, in this phylum we encounter remarkable brilliancy and variation in color. Although the carotenoids underlie the yellow, orange, red, and even blue as well as other integumentary colors of many species, there exist also conspicuous noncarotenoid pigments, for example, in shells, blood, and ink secretions among a number of forms. Moreover, by no means are all molluscs brightly colored; many, especially among the gastropods, have a dark, melanistic integument, as in some of the turbans, littorines, and abalones of California shores, wherein the exposed mantle integument is deep black.

We shall accord space here to but three of the five molluscan classes, namely the gastropods (snails, whelks, slugs), bivalves (clams, mussels, oysters), and cephalopods (octopus, squid).

Nearly a century ago, in the early 1880s, French and German workers such as de Merejkowski and Kruckenberg reported their observations of red and yellow pigments, undoubtedly carotenoids judging from their chemical behavior, in many molluscan species. De Merejkowski, for example, reported a red pigment which he first called "tetronerythrine," and later "zoonerythrine," in 117 species of invertebrates, finding rich amounts of the colored material in bryozoans, echinoderms, molluscs, and crustaceans. Of two contemporaries during the same year, Kruckenberg found yellow carotenoids in the "liver" of the European land snail *Helix pomatia,* and McMunn detected a "lutein" pigment in the carotenoid-rich digestive diverticulum of the cosmopolitan bay mussel *Mytilus edulis,* which is further discussed below.

In the latter part of 1938, Ernest Baldwin and I examined, at Cambridge, the livers of *Helix pomatia* specimens which had sealed their shell opercula while enduring a 6-month storage at temperatures of about 2° to 3°C without food. While but little greenish material, characteristic of chlorophyll degradation products, was observed in extracts of the liver, a pair of carotenes emerged, including *a*-carotene; some xanthophyllic material also was present. Earlier investigations by European workers had likewise yielded, from livers of the same species fed upon green leaves and subsequently starved for forty days, a couple of green chlorophyll-degradation fractions, as well as some carotene and xanthophyll material.

The Swedish zoologist Lönnberg, between 1931 and 1935, made preliminary observations on carotenoids of more than eighty molluscan species, including forty-one bivalves, thirty-three gastropods, three cephalopods, three amphineurans, and a scaphopod (tooth shell). In general, the digestive gland or so-called liver, the ripe ova, and in some species the skin were relatively rich in the pigments.

Yet intensive researches upon molluscan carotenoids have been rather few. Earlier studies concentrated on the red ovaries of certain bivalves, with some attention paid also to the liver and other tissues of gastropods and cephalopods.

The ripe sexual glands of the scallops *Pectunculus glycymeris* and *Pecten maximus* and of the sea mussel *Mytilus californianus* have received special study. A prominent red, oxygenated carotenoid, glycymerin, possibly identical with pectenolone, was recovered from *P. glycymeris;* and from *Pecten maximus,* was isolated another red, dihydroxy, highly unsaturated xanthophyll, pectenoxanthin. This same compound is suspected also in the red gonads of the mussel *Volsella modiolus.*

Astaxanthin reportedly is recoverable from the gastropod *Pleurobranchus elegans,* and from the red tissues of a scallop-like bivalve *Lima excavata.*

While oysters (*Ostrea*) may supply enough vitamin A to offset the lack of it in experimental animals, oyster tissues in general are poor in colored carotenoids, save perhaps in the digestive gland. Considering the diet of finely particulate organic detritus which serves largely as food for bivalves, it would be of interest to know whether the oyster is capable of deriving its vitamin A from the minor fractions of carotene in its food, as birds and mammals do.

Early studies by B. T. Scheer on the carotenoids of the large, orange-fleshed sea mussel *Mytilus californianus* afforded the first evidence of this mollusc's ability to transform zeaxanthin (or a xanthophyll closely like it) from marine algae into a new, acidic pigment, mytiloxanthin. Minor amounts of some other unique xanthophylls also were encountered, as well as pentaxanthin and fucoxanthin, known in seaweeds and other algae. The actual tissues of *Mytilus* seemed to be lacking in carotenes, which were, however, not surprisingly detected, in the gut of mussels having recently eaten. Female gonadal and somatic tissues were some twofold richer in carotenoids than corresponding parts from the male *Mytilus*.

S. Campbell found the same range of carotenoids in *M. edulis,* the cosmopolitan bay mussel, and in *M. californianus,* occurring on open shores of the Pacific Coast of North Ameriica. She reported alloxanthin, a newer, highly unsaturated derivative of zeaxanthin, to be the predominant carotenoid present; she also confirmed Scheer's report of mytiloxanthin, and listed several other xanthophylls stored by the mussels.

Certain crustaceans, parasitic or commensal in mussels, were also studied. The parasitic copepod *Mytilicola intestinalis,* found in the alimentary tract and digestive gland of *M. edulis,* appears red due to the presence of hemoglobin. No carotene, echinenone, isocryptoxanthin, or canthaxanthin are stored by this parasite, but astaxanthin and esters thereof were found stored by females.

A harmless commensal crustacean is the round-bodied, so-called pea crab, *Pinnotheres pisum.* Females reside in the mantle cavity of *M. edulis,* exhibit red ovaries, and are much larger than the males. The three most abundant carotenoids commonly found in this commensal crustacean are β-carotene (30 percent), alloxanthin (29 percent), and lutein (22 percent), giving a total of 81 percent of all carotenoids observed; echine-none (6 percent), canthaxanthin (4 percent), and esterified asta-xanthin (4 percent) aggregated all save 5 percent of the rest. This pea crab, being commensal as mentioned, does not actu-ally parasitize its host, but consumes an identical carotenoid-supplying diet, including single-celled phytoplankton, small zooplankton, and leptopel, or finely suspended organic matter. It may well be imagined that the resident crab receives the aggre-gate regime in "packets" or ropes of the mixed materials incor-porated in the host's mucus, elaborated for making such collec-tions. As a result of this activity, the visitant would appear to assume more the role of a harpy, stealing food en route to the mussel's mouth, rather than being cast as a flesh-eating predator.

Certain gastropod molluscs carry rich stores of carotenoids, in numerous instances conjugated with protein, and giving vari-ous blue, violet, or other colors, as in the case of some sea stars.

The South American land gastropod *Pila* is known to deposit highly pigmented egg masses, usually red in color, though in some species green. Eggs of the Argentine species *P. glauca* yield their carotenoid chromoprotein to water. Denaturation liberates deep orange carotenoid material in solution, resolvable into six or more different fractions, chiefly hypophasic, and therefore oxygenated.

An herbivorous freshwater snail, *Pomacea canaliculata australis,* concocts, with its egg jelly, a red astaxanthin-glyco-protein complex—ovorubin—which has an impressive molecu-lar weight of 330,000, and exhibits spectral maxima in the green region, at 510 and 545 nm in aqueous media. The chromopro-tein demonstrates relatively high stability against denaturation by heat (below 100°C), by cold alkali, and by adsorption to solid surfaces. Nor is it readily attacked by the protein-splitting enzyme trypsin; in fact, it actually inhibits tryptic digestion. Moreover, the chromoprotein has been observed to remain immune from attack by substantial populations of bacteria and molds while exposed thereto for a year's duration at 5°C and pH 6.

The pronounced immunity of this carotenoid-protein complex to thermal, chemical, or adsorptive denaturation, as well as against degradation by microbial or other proteases, plus its ability to conserve imbibed water during exposure of the snail's eggs to warm air at the edges of pools—all suggest a striking degree of biochemical adaptation for survival in this species.

Far and away the most beautifully colored molluscs, perhaps of all animals, are found among the marine chromodorid nudibranch slugs (pls. 23-24). Watery extracts of their blue, purple, pink, or violet integumentary pigments, all chromoproteins, turn pink or orange when the protein moiety of the complex has been denatured by heating or by immersion in alcohol. In the nudibranchs, the natural yellow, orange, or red spots, stripes, or other integumentary patches reflect the presence of carotenoids associated with lipid or fatty deposits, or possibly dissolved in the lipoprotein portion. Such pigments therefore cannot be leached away, as are the chromoproteins, by mere soaking in tap water or other foreign aqueous media.

It has perhaps come as a surprise to some that, despite the arresting beauty and brilliance of their pigmentation, numbers of these nudibranch species are not among the innovators that derive previously unanticipated compounds from conventional chemical precursors. As a point of fact, they reveal a remarkable lack of originality in this regard, discounting their ability to conjugate certain ready-made, polar dietary carotenoids with proteins, resulting in a spectacular display of color (incidentally unseen by them). Unlike many other animals, including representatives from coelenterates, arthropods, echinoderms, and even some fishes and birds, these carnivorous marine slugs seem chiefly to assimilate and store, molecularly unchanged (save for the ligation to proteins), carotenoids preexistent in their prey, including notably sedentary forms such as hydroids, bryozoans, and sponges.

J. W. McBeth (mentioned earlier in the Preface) studied the carotenoids of several highly colorful nudibranch species, including *Hopkinsia rosacea* (pl. 23) (of a delicate, overall pink color), the purple-skinned, orange-gilled slug *Flabellinopsis iodinea* (pl. 24), and the slugs *Anisodoris nobilis* (orange to light yellow), *Dendrodoris fulva* (yellow to yellow-orange), and

Doriopsilla albopunctata (dark brown); both of these latter species display small white spots over the dorsal surface, as suggested by the specific designation of the last-named.

The latter three are known to store about one-fifth of their total carotenoids as the rare aromatic compound isorenieratene (App., 28), encountered also in certain bacteria and sponges. Each of the slugs was unusual also in storing substantial fractions of a- and β-carotenes, *Anisodoris* yielding 21 percent a- and 23 percent β-carotene; *Dendrodoris* 15.5 percent and 42 percent respectively; and *Doriopsilla* 7 percent and 25 percent. Another nudibranch, *Triopha carpenteri* (with deep-orange areas on white-to-pale-yellow skin) stored no carotenes whatever, but manufactured more than half its xanthophyllic pigments as trophioxanthin. The latter was newly found and named by McBeth, and was found to share some characteristics with hopkinsiaxanthin. The three bryozoan species comprising the prey of *Triopha* were discovered as yielding many carotenoid fractions, seven of which match exactly the respective fractions discovered in the predatory slug. Moreover, the prominent carotenoid from the bryozoan extract was indeed triophioxanthin, the principal one detected in the skin of the consumer.

Hopkinsia, rich in skin carotenoids, yields several fractions, 70 percent of the total of which appears to be hopkinsiaxanthin, a rare orange pigment of exceptional chemical structure (App., 26). Here again, this is also the principal carotenoid stored by the pink, encrusting bryozoan *Eurystomella bilabiata,* the slug's chief prey.

A singular instance may be found in the purple slug *Flabellinopsis* (pl. 24), which bears astaxanthin as the only carotenoid; this is traceable also to its principal prey, the hydroid *Eudendrium ramosum.* The pair of reddish rhinophores, or hornlike, fleshy projections from the head yielded two esters along with the uncombined compound. Also, free astaxanthin, representing 80 percent of the total fractions present in the orange-colored cerata, or fingerlike gills over the dorsal body surface, was accompanied by two esters of the same compound. The ripe, pink egg masses, readily visible through the blue-violet skin, carried only free astaxanthin, often encountered in other marine invertebrate ova. Finally, the blue-violet skin pigment was shown to be a protein-conjugated astaxanthin.

Turning briefly to the cephalopods, the octopods and deca-pods (squids) are recognized as forms capable of exhibiting rapid and marked color changes involving their outer integu-ment. These colors may vary from pale yellow-brown through tan, to an even darker brown or deep-chocolate color. Some octopus species may assume an overall transient red color. None of these observed colors are due to carotenoids; melanins and certain other nitrogenous, water-miscible pigments are responsible.

The decapods *Sepiola scandica, Rossia macrosoma, Eledone cirrosa,* and *Loligo opalescens* failed to yield significant amounts of carotenoids from any tissues save for traces of xan-thophyllic material from the eyes (and somewhat more from the "liver" of *Eledone,* which produced an orange-yellow extract in acetone). The unripe ovaries and clear, hyaline eggs of *Sepiola* lacked carotenoids. The two-spotted octopus or devilfish, *Octo-pus bimaculatus,* of the Southern California coast, likewise yields but little carotenoid, whether from skin, muscle, bran-chial hearts, pericardial glands, or salivary glands (which secrete the venom), but may carry copious amounts in the large liver (hepatopancreas, or digestive gland), and moderate but surprising concentrations in the *ink.*

The large liver-pancreas gland yields carotenoids correspond-ing with those ingested in the diet, including carotenes, xantho-phylls—both free and esterified, and very frequently astaxan-thin, derived by the predator from its crustacean food.

What arrested our attention was the discovery of carotenoids, secreted from the ink gland into the dark, melanin-rich ink. Moreover, only xanthophylls, partly free, partly esterified, were recognized there, including the familiar acidogenic member; carotenes proper never were detected in the viscous fluid (Fox and Crane, cited by Fox, 1976).

Concentrations of carotenoids in livers (plus attached ink sac and contents) of wild specimens varied from about 1.2 to 28.3 mg per 100 g of fresh tissue, whereas the ink had less, varying between 0.55 and 2.00 mg per 100 g. The recoverable ink would constitute no more than about 6 percent of the total weight of liver, attached ink sac, and ink proper.

S. C. Crane (also mentioned in the Preface) pursued the octopus liver-carotenoid problem further. It had been determined that carotenoids disappear from both liver and ink when the animal is denied food for a time. Crane showed, moreover, that this mollusc, like man, the common frog, and a few other non-selectors, is itself nondiscriminating as to assimilation and storage of carotenoids in its hepatopancreas, where 95 percent or more of them are to be found; here it is present in carotenes, free or esterified xanthophylls, or astaxanthin. Crane demonstrated this by feeding captive specimens for about four weeks each on appropriate diets. When fed carotenoid-free flesh (hog liver or heart) *Octopus* lost all of the stored carotenoid material. On a diet of flesh carrying only carotenes (horse liver) or only xanthophylls (in bright orange or yellow skin, covering the white flesh of Garibaldi, the marine goldfish) or solely astaxanthin in the hypoderm of the large local crayfish or "spiny lobster," *Panulirus interruptus* (pl. 18), the respective consumers readily assimilated any such carotenoids into the liver, but no carotenes were detected in the ink of those animals fed on horse liver.

The liver-pancreas of cephalopods is a relatively fatty organ, containing as much as 7 to 14 percent of total lipids on a wet-weight basis. The chief physiological role here seems to be secretory, generating digestive enzymes which are then transmitted through ducts into the gut during feeding.

The secretion of xanthophylls into the ink gland, and thence into the ink, later to be discharged into the water via the ink duct, likens the physiological process to a limited number of others, including the transfer and storage of carotenoids in egg yolk by many animals, the secretion of such pigments into honey and wax by bees, and into milk fat from mammary glands, as well as into crop milk created by some birds, such as flamingos, for nourishment of the chicks. There are also somewhat parallel processes of carotenoid discharge via secretion in other animals, for example, sloughing of the epidermis in general, discharge of earwax in cattle, the elaboration of feathers, many of which are richly pigmented with these compounds, and the voiding of yellow carotenoids in waxy kernels from the ventral, femoral skin pits of certain iguanas.

ARTHROPODS

Crustaceans

It is likely that animals of this phylum may have received wider attention, even respecting their colors, than most other invertebrate groups. This would apply especially to the two classes Crustacea and Insecta, not only because of the variety and brilliance of their colors, but particularly in view of the enormous numbers of species, their worldwide distribution, and, ultimately, the economic significance of many forms, whether serving as food from the sea (shrimps, lobsters, crabs, etc.), or *in* the sea. Microcrustaceans such as copepods and euphausiids are by far the most numerous of all marine animals, and constitute the primary food of many other, larger animals, for example, many fish species, and certain whales, which consume tons of krill. Though by no means least, the importance to man of beneficial as well as many harmful insects is well-established.

Many are familiar with the various shades of purple, blue, bright and subdued green colors, and diverse tones of brown or gray commonly observed in bodies and eggs of numerous crustaceans. Heating or preserving in alcohol, or even in formaldehyde, releases the colored pigments as the proteins are denatured. In many species the dominant color is light or dark red, even orange, although the carotenoid is in all probability conjugated with protein, or, as the author recently discovered, chemically joined to chitin, the tough, nitrogenous polysaccharide of the crustacean exoskeleton. Chitin-conjugated astaxanthin is of a dark-red color, similar to that of the carotenoid itself, in the red, sometimes purplish-red carapace or exoskeleton of the kelp-eating crab *Taliepus nuttallii* (pl. 19). Three other polar carotenoids that accompany the chief pigment (which constitutes nearly 80 percent of all fractions) as conjugants to the chitinous armor of this crab are echinenone, phoenicoxanthin, and canthaxanthin (App., 19a, 20, and 21).

Taliepus, subsisting mainly on seaweeds, doubtless converts the β-carotene, and perhaps some of the algal xanthophylls, into stores of ketonic carotenoids carried firmly joined to the material of its skeleton.

One of the most colorful crustaceans is the American lobster of commerce, *Homarus americanus,* which usually displays an all-over dark-green color, but may sometimes bear a variegated livery, wherein green is interspersed with black, red, blue, cream-spotted, or calico patterns. There are photographic records of such harlequin lobster specimens, some manifesting an arresting, bizarre, pied appearance, being colored a normal, dark green along one exact half of the body's length, including the head end, claw, walking-legs, body carapace, and telson, or fanlike tail, and of a uniformly bright orange color over the whole of the opposite half, with a sharp, median line of demarcation along the entire length. Such a manifestation must reflect a bilateral metabolic pattern originating in the embryonic two-cell stage.

An attractive, oceanic, rafting crustacean is the blue goose-barnacle *Lepas fascicularis,* the striking coloration of whose inner and outer body tissues and of its ripe eggs is due to the presence, as in other species, of protein-conjugated astaxanthin.

Lepas is a small, stalked barnacle, borne at the sea surface by its own mature float, or when younger by attaching its stalk's end to free-floating objects, such as the siphonophore *Velella lata,* bits of wood or cork, lumps of tar, or sizable feathers afloat at sea. During a continuing onshore wind, these barnacles, along with countless *Velella,* may be wafted in and deposited at the tidal edge of the beach.

Relative concentrations of astaxanthin in *Lepas* tissues vary, from the content of ripe, blue eggs (5 mg per 100 g) to whole gut (2 mg per 100 g) and other body tissues, including immature eggs (ca. 1 mg per 100 g). In these loci, astaxanthin indeed has been measured at 93 percent, 56 percent, and 82 percent, respectively, while there are occasional minor proportions of β-carotene in somatic tissues, and esterified zeaxanthinlike material in all tissues.

It has been suggested that the binding of astaxanthin to protein may serve to stabilize both members of the complex against damage by either heat or excessive light in the warm, exposed oceanic habitat of the barnacle (cf. ovorubin in the exposed eggs of the snail *Pomacea*). Also, the conjugated linkage may implement a higher concentration of the carotenoid than might otherwise be accommodated, for instance, in mere oil droplets, wherein it might be less readily available. A parallel degree of chemical stabilization of the astaxanthin itself as a protein conjugant might serve the organism in processes of development and growth or in other ways.

Ovoverdin, the green astaxanthin protein of lobster eggs, persists unchanged until shortly before the eggs hatch, when the protein moiety is detached, liberating free astaxanthin.

In such a connection it is interesting to recall that astaxanthin is present in the eyes of many crustaceans and some insects; indeed many copepods have been found to store major amounts of their vitamin A supplies therein, often along with β-carotene. Inasmuch as vitamin A is directly involved in the biochemistry of vision itself, it has been particularly interesting to note that many small crustaceans, including certain amphipods, isopods, cladocerans, and even some copepods, lack vitamin A, and yet have prominent eyes carrying astaxanthin, whether in its usual red form or in the blue, protein-conjugated state. It may be that this widely occurring carotenoid plays some part in light perception (whether or not there might be a truly visual function) in some eyed invertebrate species, recalling the suspected light perception in sea stars equipped with blue astaxanthin-protein "eye spots" or optic cushions at the end of each ray.

Other crustaceans known to assimilate β-carotene, converting it internally to astaxanthin, are the prawns *Penaeus japonicus* and *Metapenaeus barbata*. The crab *Portunus trituberculatus* and the spiny "lobster" *Panulirus japonicus,* a marine crayfish, convert dietary β-carotene internally to isocryptoxanthin and its direct ketone derivative, echinenone, while in the hypodermis they also generate canthaxanthin, astaxanthin, and allied intermediate derivatives.

A degenerate crustacean, *Sacculina carcina,* is parasitic at various sites on the body of its host crab *Carcinus meanas,* of European coasts. The marauder seems to be highly selective in robbing its host of carotenoids; of the many types available at different sites, including even the hepatopancreas, rich in varieties and quantities of carotenoids, only β-carotene is assimilated by the parasitic *Sacculina*.

Shore isopod species of the genus *Idotea* have been found to exhibit considerable flexibility in adapting their chromatic appearance to match the colors of plants and other background features of their immediate surroundings. Some species can effect the proportions of red, green, and brown pigmentation of their external surfaces rather rapidly. They do this by varying the relative amounts of carotenoid, notably canthaxanthin, in uncombined state (red or orange) or conjugated with protein, giving green complexes, while various ratios of the two factors afford shades of brown.

W. L. Lee and B. Gilchrist have worked, individually and as collaborators, on the pigments of several of these marine crustaceans, including a study of the little gray, sand-burrowing shrimp *Emerita analoga*,* which feeds upon small algal plants and marine detrital particles which are lodged in the sand from each receding wave. *Emerita* utilizes β-carotene for generating echinenone, canthaxanthin, and astaxanthin, in that order of sequence. The chief carotenoid stored is astaxanthin, amounting to some 45 percent of the total, while zeaxanthin, second in prominence, is accompanied by minor amounts of algal xanthophylls and very little β-carotene. The seasonal excess of astaxanthin in eggs and carapace parallels steep rises in exposure to sunlight and to elevated temperatures of the sea surface. Thus astaxanthin may likely serve both adults and eggs as a screen against thermal and light rays potentially injurious to protein, and may also aid the developing young in their stabilization and conservation of protein food reserves.

Insects

Many examples within this class of arthropods owe their rich pigmentation to the presence of carotenoids. We shall consider but a relatively few for comparative purposes.

---

*One of my assistants (L-G) has enjoyed exposing some of these little, roundish, so-called sand crabs to gently boiling water, thus denaturing the protein and conferring a pink, astaxanthin color to the whole carapace and legs; she then removed and cooled the bodies, placed them in a suitable container, and asked graduate students or young faculty biologists for an identification of her "discovery."

The honeybee *Apis mellifera* owes the reddish, orange, or yellow colors of various honeys largely to the presence of carotenoids, derived from the species of pollen consumed. Certain carotenoids from the same sources are present in propolis (bee glue), which the insects transform into the wax of their honeycombs. β-Carotene is a pigment characteristic of honey, while extracts of wax itself have yielded four carotenoid fractions encountered in the propolis precursor. The fractions include β-carotene and an ester of lutein.

Other hymenopteran insects yielding carotenoids include certain species of ants which deposit the pigments in their eggs. The yellow body colors of wasps and hornets, however, are due to the presence of a completely different kind of pigment—the pterins, which are discussed in later pages.

Green, blue, and blue-green strains of caterpillar of the clouded sulfur butterfly *Colias philodice,* a pest in alfalfa and clover fields, are interesting from the viewpoint of the degree to which their respective body colors affect their survival. Blue mutants fail to assimilate carotenoids from their plant food and, when developed into adults, lay colorless eggs from which hatch blue- or blue-green-colored larvae. Adult females of the green variety, however, deposit yellow eggs, reflecting the presence of carotenoids absorbed from the food. Caterpillars hatching from these eggs combine the yellow pigmentary color with their natural blue component, therefore appearing green, and consequently enjoying a high degree of protective coloration against their natural background of green clover or alfalfa. The blue-colored caterpillars, on the other hand, inherit a recessive factor that leads to the oxidative destruction of dietary carotene (or to its nonassimilation). Thus they are conspicuous against their green background, and hence more readily seen and devoured by English sparrows.

A small parasitic wasp, *Apanteles flaviconchae,* preying on the green *Colias* caterpillar, assimilates the latter's carotenoids and ultimately creates cocoons of golden-yellow silk, whereas individuals which have preyed instead upon the blue-green genotype of caterpillar spin cocoons of white silk.

Another small wasp, *Microgaster conglomeratus,* parasitizes the caterpillar of the white butterfly *Pieris brassicae,* deriving from its lymph, skin, and intestine a mixture of a-carotene and taraxanthin, which subsequently are deposited in and color the silk of the predator's cocoon.

Production of astaxanthin is represented among this general group of animals in certain mites (arachnids), the potato beetle *Leptinotarsa decemlineata,* and the rose-colored locust *Schisto-cerca gregaria,* in addition to the migratory locust *Locusta migratoria migratorioides,* which derives β-carotene, out of which it generates astaxanthin, from a diet solely of grass. At sexual maturity, β-carotene in the fat droplets replaces the hypodermal astaxanthin. Astaxanthin is however present in the eyes of both immature and adult locusts, while fatty tissues and gonads of both sexes are pigmented by β-carotene and traces of a-carotene but lack xanthophylls.

Newly laid locust eggs contain β-carotene as the only pigment; this, during incubation, is converted gradually to astaxanthin through an oxidative process. Although locusts manifest no preformed vitamin A, they store β-carotene in amounts sufficient to render the insect a chosen dietary component among some people. It is worthy of notice that, while the embryo locust is without vitamin A, and whereas the β-carotene has been converted quantitatively into astaxanthin and stored in the eyes among other sites, the young hoppers apparently have sight upon hatching. This fact contributes to the suspicion that, in this insect, as well as in many small marine crustaceans similarly equipped, the ocular astaxanthin, perhaps combined with protein, may serve as a rudimentary photosensitive system. This leads to the possibility of reaction toward incident light, even if the mechanism fails to confer complete vision as does the system of vitamin A protein, or retinaldehyde-opsin-conjugated protein in vertebrate eyes.

Yellow-blooded caterpillars of the silk moth *Bombyx mori* secrete yellow cocoon silk, while genetic variants containing no blood carotenoids spin white silk. If *Bombyx* is to produce yellow silk, it must possess hereditary factors controlling: (1) the capacity for assimilating the consumed carotenoids, (2) the ability to spare the carotenoid from metabolic oxidation, and (3) a facility for secreting the carotenoid via the serigenous gland into the silk as this is manufactured. The yellow silk of *B. mori* yields identifiable lutein (App., 7), taraxanthin (App., 11), and violaxanthin (App., 12) among the carotenoids derived from the caterpillar's consumption of its mulberry-leaf diet. Xanthophylls preponderate greatly over carotenes in the cocoon silk, for example, in ratios of 24 to only about 0.7 mg per 100 g, or some 35 to 1.

Many beetles offer striking examples of typical carotenoid pigmentation, notably over the exposed surfaces of their hard elytra or wing covers. The lady beetle *Coccinella septempunctata* (pl. 33), bearing seven black, melanistic spots on the bright red background, yields a- and β-carotenes, lycopene (App., 5) and/or γ-carotene (App., 3) and sometimes minor fractions of xanthophylls. Such beetles are, of course, not plant eaters, but carnivores, preying upon plant-sucking aphids, whence their pigments are derived secondhand.

As we proceed from our brief survey of the carotenoids among the arthopod phylum, we should take passing note of a recent finding of red carotenoid stores in a representative of yet another class, the Arachnoidea, subclass Merostomata, order Xiphosura. The animal of reference is the so-called king crab or horseshoe crab (which is not indeed a crab), *Limulus polyphemus,* common in shallow, quiet waters of the Atlantic coast from Maine south to Yucatan. This hard-shelled, thorny, literally sword-tailed creature, predatory upon shellfish generally, has a brick-red coxal gland, a bilateral, eight-lobed organ, embedded in the muscles about the base of the second, third, fourth, and fifth legs, and performing an excretory function analogous to that of a nephridium or renal gland. E. G. Ball has given some study to the carotenoid pigments present in the gland, as well as those in the eggs, hepatopancreas, and blood amebocytes of this arachnoid.

Glands weighing from 250 to 1350 mg (wet), recovered from 21 adult animals (11 females and 10 males) showed a carotenoid content of from 25 to 226 μg per g, with an average value of 111 μg/g wet tissue. About seven chromatographic fractions were recovered, including β-carotene, echinenone (App., 19a), two hydroxycarotenoids, and possibly a fraction of phoenicopterone (App., 19b) ($=$ 4-keto-a-carotene).

Other tissues mentioned above yielded lower concentrations

of carotenoids. Prominent fractions of egg carotenoids and of those from amebocytes corresponded with those encountered in the coxal gland, while β-carotene was the only type definitely identifiable in the hepatopancreas extract. The latter organ, a very large one, carries the major quantity of carotenoid material, at a level of about 31 $\mu g/g$. There has been no indication of a site where conversion of β-carotene—stored in the hepatopancreas—into oxygenated derivatives might occur; it would appear nevertheless manifest that the animal manages the oxidation in some manner. The problem calls for additional study.

CHORDATES

Among the primitive (nonvertebrate) chordates are numbered the tunicates, or ascidians, alternatively so named because they are invested with a kind of cloak or tunic, and because the general overall shape is saclike, thus from *askos* [Gk., "sac or bladder"].

Among these—the only group whose pigments have received serious attention—bright colors occur in some of the free-swimming forms, though not commonly. Among sessile ascidians, known commonly as sea squirts, from their shape and habit of ejecting a stream of water when suddenly contracting, there are both solitary and colonial representatives, many of which are brilliantly pigmented; still the group as a whole is not prominent or readily available for study. The pigments of these striking but primitive and degenerate animals of the chordate phylum have therefore received less study than that focused upon members of both higher and lower varieties.

Colored species of simple ascidians rich in carotenoids are *Ascidia virginica, Styela rustica,* and *Corella parallelograma,* while *Molgula occulta* and the common greenish sea squirt *Ciona intestinalis* yield but scarce carotenoid material. Some colonial species giving richly colored extracts are *Synoicium (Amoroucium) pulmonaria, Botryllus schlosseri,* and *Maxilla mammilaris.*

Some ascidians given special attention by Lederer included two solitary forms, *Halocynthia papillosa* and *Microcosmus sulcatus,* the so-called "social" ascidian *Dendrodoa grossularia,* attached to its neighbors at the base, and *Botryllus schlosseri.*

Halocynthia, characterized by a dark-red tunic and orange-colored internal organs, yielded a rich quantity of astaxanthin and secondary amounts of cynthiaxanthin, resembling, but not identical with, zeaxanthin. There were also mere traces of β-carotene.

From *Microcosmus* major yields of free xanthophylls and a ketone suspected to be echinenone were recovered, along with a-carotene. One of the xanthophylls resembled zeaxanthin, another lutein. The esterified fractions were suspected to be fucoxanthin, the chief carotenoid of marine brown algae.

The violet-red or rose-colored social tunicate *Dendrodoa* contained rich stores of astaxanthin, some traces of esterified xanthophylls, and minor amounts of β- and a-carotenes.

The brown-red compound ascidian *Botryllus* was found to be variable in its carotenoid stores. There appeared to be major proportions of xanthophylls, with only minor quantities of β-carotene and another fraction reminiscent of lycopene, the prominent red hydrocarbon of tomatoes. Of the xanthophylls recovered, variable proportions of capsanthin (App., 25), capsorubin, pectenoxanthin, and a fourth unfamiliar fraction were encountered. Lederer suggested that the inconsistently encountered capsanthin and capsorubin fractions might well reflect the consumption, by these filter-feeding animals, of finely particulate pimiento wastes (rich in the two red compounds) discharged with other kitchen refuse into the harbor habitat of the animal colonies.

Fishes

This animal class has long enjoyed outstanding distinction among vertebrates owing to the display of bright coloration and varied patterns. The members are, indeed, rivaled in this regard by only one other vertebrate class—the birds, many of which exhibit equally arresting chromatic brilliance, notably in their feathers.

Many published studies have dealt with the carotenoids of fishes, but we shall consider here only a representative few. It may be stated at the outset that by far the commonest carotenoid incident in the fishes is the light-yellow xanthophyll tunaxanthin or 3,3'-dihydroxy- ϵ -carotene (App., 10), studied and first characterized by some Japanese workers, and more recently by G. F. Crozier and D. W. Wilkie at La Jolla. Tunaxanthin indeed is, beyond doubt, the precise compound mistaken in earlier days by many of us for taraxanthin or lutein, both of which exhibit absorption spectra closely resembling that of the carotenoid named, but from which separation can be effected only on a critically chosen chromatographic plate. Zeaxanthin, an earlier recognized xanthophyll, is also of fairly common incidence among fishes.

The rich deposits of astaxanthin in the liver of the ribbon-bodied oarfish *Regalicus glesne,* in that of the lumper or lumpsucker *Cyclopterus lumpus,* and in the skin and muscle of both *Salmo* and *Oncorhyncus* species of salmon, have long been acknowledged and assumed to derive from the fishes' consumption of various small crustaceans.

The marine dorado *Beryx decadactylus* and the red genotype of the common goldfish *Carassius auratus* store much astaxanthin in the skin; *Beryx* exhibits the same red compound also in the mucus of mouth and gills, as well as in the sclera and iris of its eyes. In the goldfish, whose stores of astaxanthin indeed are chiefly in the skin, this prominent carotenoid is accompanied by minor fractions of neutral xanthophylls and even traces of carotenes. There are some differences in carotenoid content evident between the red and yellow genotypes of *Carassius.* Red extracts from the fins of the red variant yield astaxanthin as the chief fraction, with secondary amounts of neutral xanthophylls, while fins of the yellow variety give golden-yellow extracts of neutral xanthophylls accompanied by but questionable traces of astaxanthin.

There are fish species which store no astaxanthin, or store it inconsistently. The freshwater perch *Perca fluviatilis* yields only neutral xanthophylls; the pike *Esox lucius,* possessing red fins, also the eelpout *Lota lota,* bearing yellow-spotted skin, likewise seem to store no astaxanthin among their xanthophylls. The sunfish *Orthagoriscus mola* yields but traces of astaxanthin from its very fatty liver, and the liver of one of the angler fishes, *Lophius piscatorius,* the goosefish, contains but little of the commonly found red, acidogenic carotenoid.

The skin of the brown trout *Salmo trutta* commonly stores considerable proportions of astaxanthin among its carotenoids. This is controlled experimentally by feeding captive trout rich sources of the pigment, such as fresh salmon ova.

Professor F. B. Sumner and I in our early work together, determined that several species of marine fish deposit no carotenes, nor astaxanthin, but only esterified xanthophylls, in the integument and fins; the chief compound was believed at the time to be taraxanthin, but almost certainly was indeed tunaxanthin, so commonly found in fishes.

The species studied were the Pacific killifish *Fundulus parvipinnis,* the greenfish or opaleye *Girella nigricans,* the longjawed goby *Gillichthys mirabilis,* and the Garibaldi or marine goldfish *Hypsypops rubicunda* mentioned earlier (pl. 13).

Fundulus not only stored the xanthophyll fed to it, but was found to be capable of converting dietary carotene into the kind of xanthophyll stored. Some experiments on color adaptation showed that *Fundulus* maintained in matte white containers gradually became very pale; when kept over the same period in yellow-colored aquariums, they became bright yellow in overall body color, whereas specimens maintained in red surroundings finally assumed a ruddy-brown livery (from visible blood vessels against a brown, melanin background); and the specimens exposed to black bowls became so inky black, during the same span of time, as to render them well-nigh invisible against their background.

Amid such color changes, two potential factors were alleged to be operative. Pale fishes from the white background had maximally contracted the pigment masses within their black melanophores and yellow xanthophores, thus leaving the aggregate impression of whiteness; fishes which reacted to living in a yellow milieu maximally dispersed the pigment within their xanthophores (without altering the actual *quantities* present), while managing to keep the melanin within their melanophores maximally contracted into a small, central mass in the center of each such cell; and those fishes who occupied only a black environment, though preserving the yellow-pigmented bodies within their xanthophores, succeeded in keeping the latter maximally contracted, while spreading the melanosomes within the black cells into their full dendritic outlines. Indeed, these fishes may also, like the little guppy, *Lebistes reticulatus* of freshwaters, have responded to protracted residence in a black-walled, black-bottomed aquarium by actually implementing an increase in the numbers of melanophores, hence augmenting the total quantities of integumentary melanin, as well as according the included pigment maximal spreading.

Notwithstanding these striking color contrasts, however, analysis of the fishes' skins for total xanthophyll concentration following residence of a month or two on their respective backgrounds (though while on a common diet) disclosed no significant difference among the four sets. Nor did residence of *Fundulus* in total darkness for six weeks (always on the same, adequate food) effect any changes in concentrations of xanthophyll esters as found by analysis of the skin.

The marine goldfish *Hypsypops,* bearing specular, shining blue spots as a juvenile (pl. 14), and changing to a brilliant orange-colored coat when adult (pl. 13), shows quantitative increases in its integumentary xanthophyll esters with increasing age (weight), undergoing a fourfold increase, from 6 to 24 mg per 100 g as the animal's weight increases from a total of 60 to 500 g.

Hypsypops is not able, as is *Fundulus,* to oxidize dietary carotene to a xanthophyll, but, on a diet containing carotene as the only carotenoid, *Hypsypops,* again in contrast to *Fundulus,* finally is able to assimilate traces of carotene itself into the skin.

The goby *Gillichthys mirabilis,* maintained, as was *Fundulus,* upon backgrounds of different colors, exhibited similar matching changes in color; again, like *Fundulus,* the goby showed no significant changes in the concentrations of xanthophyll esters in its skin. *Gillichthys* is suspectedly capable of converting carotene into xanthophylls.

Similar experiments with the greenfish *Girella nigricans* involved small, sexually immature specimens in both chromatic and dietary studies (larger, adult members of this species are incompatible among themselves when placed in aquariums of limited dimensions, lacking hiding places). When maintained in white, yellow, red, or black aquariums the young *Girella* manifested color changes of the same general character as had been observed in adults of the other two species. *Girella,* however, revealed an arresting lability of its integumentary carotenoids; each of the experimental batches underwent decreases in the concentration of their carotenoids. This loss was much accelerated, for some reason, in fishes held in *white* containers, while residence on yellow or on neutral gray backgrounds delayed the loss appreciably, suggesting an effect of background *shade* or reflecting capacity rather than actual color. The specimens residing in the black containers lost their skin carotenoids least readily. In all experiments on all three species of fish, the *incident* light from above was of the same intensity, with only the reflected fraction differing; the *albedo,* or ratio of reflected to incident light intensity, thus would appear to be a direct factor in the ability of this species to maintain the integrity of its supplies of integumentary xanthophylls.

Not all fishes advertise their carotenoid pigmentation; some species indeed lack carotenoids completely, while others may store but small amounts. In more recent work, G. F. Crozier and I have examined tissues of some less advanced fishes for carotenoids with findings as follows: of three elasmobranch species, including two sharks and a ray, the Pacific mako *Isurus glaucus* yielded no skin carotenoids, while the horned shark *Heterodontus francisci* was found to store minor concentrations of zeaxanthin esters in its skin, and more than twofold the concentration of the same xanthophyll, mostly unesterified in the liver. The thornback ray *Platyrhinoides triseriata* likewise stores only minor amounts of zeaxanthin esters in its skin, and in the liver more than 46-fold the quantity (7.86 mg/100 g), nearly all unesterified. Various species of sharks, dogfishes, skates, and rays store minor quantities of liver carotenoids, but the characteristic whole dull-gray skin carries little or none of the pigments.

We examined two specimens of the hagfish *Eptatretus stoutii,* one of which had been held captive for three months at 7°C, and the other a mere week at the same temperature. Neither liver, skin, nor eggs yielded any pigment to alcoholic extracts, and all were destitute of carotenoid material. Two lampreys, *Lampetra fluviatilis* and *L. planeri*, yielded lutein from their larval stages and from the adult skin.

Finally, the author was able to obtain materials from a rare fish, the coelacanth *Latimeria chalumnae*, taken from deep waters off Mutsamudu, Anjouan Isle, in the Comoros. Scales and liver had been preserved in formaldehyde (very probably precluding any oxidative processes) for a two-month period. Scales yielded carotenoid-free, colorless extracts, while a sizable chunk of liver (33.5 g) gave a pale, cloudy-yellow alcoholic extract, containing large quantities of fatty materials but no trace of carotenoid.

Some studies have been conducted, beyond the earlier ones relating to *Fundulus parvipinnis*, concerning the faculty of certain fishes to convert supplied carotenoids into more heavily oxygenated compounds. Crozier studied the California sheephead *Pimelometopon pulchrum*, which exhibits conspicuous sexual dimorphism and dichromatism. The adult male has a high fleshy, rounded crest extending from above the eyes, back from the head for a short way, and bears deep-black melanistic skin over the head and tail, with a broad, bright-red "saddle" between. The mature female has a symmetrical, crescent-shaped back, and is pigmented uniformly pink or red over her back and sides (pl. 16).

This unusual fish species is remarkable in several other respects. In the first place, it is a sequential hermaphrodite, in that all the young begin life as females, and remain so until about the seventh year, when some undergo the typical change in shape and coloration, assuming the characteristics of the male. Second, unlike other fishes—or most others—the sheephead stores all of its carotenoid pigment in its skin, save for mere traces in the ripe ovary and the eye; there is *none* in the liver (a rare circumstance, notably in a species storing it elsewhere), nor of course in the adult spermary. Moreover, *Pimelometopon* is able to effect a remarkable biochemical transformation of stored tunaxanthin (App., 10), probably with zeaxanthin (App., 8) as intermediary, into astaxanthin (App., 22); this conversion involves translocation of two double-bond pairs from the 4-5 to the 5-6 carbons of each terminal ring, as well as the introduction of an oxygen atom in replacement of two hydrogens, on the 4-carbon of each ring.

The juveniles, all immature females, exhibit a golden-yellow skin color, with black, melanistic spots on dorsal, pelvic, anal, and caudal fins. These spots fade as (or after) the golden phase is replaced by a bright-red coloration. The prominent carotenoid in the integument of young, freshly caught specimens is esterified tunaxanthin, amounting to nearly 60 percent of the totals, while nearly another third is esterified astaxanthin, and the negligible remainder zeaxanthin esters. Adult male skin yields no more than traces of tunaxanthin, all esterified, and varying proportions of zeaxanthin esters. Even the adult female, bearing in her skin approximately the same concentrations of total carotenoids as does the male, stores about 90 percent thereof as esterified astaxanthin, in addition to somewhat more residual tunaxanthin than is carried by the male. Ovaries yield but traces of pigment, all of it free zeaxanthin.

Japanese workers have demonstrated the ability of the goldfish *Carassius auratus* to oxidize lutein to its 4-keto derivative and similarly to transform zeaxanthin readily, and β-carotene also to a slight extent, into astaxanthin, while echinenone and canthaxanthin were not found to be thus metabolized when fed to the species. The skin carotenoids in *Carassius* seem to comprise nearly equal fractions of esterified astaxanthin (45.5 percent) and esterified 4-ketolutein (41 percent), while the remaining fractions include esters of zeaxanthin and of lutein, as well as minor proportions of free phoenixocanthin and traces of uncombined astaxanthin.

As *Carassius* grows from its dark-gray-skinned juvenile phase, gradually attaining the fully developed, orange-colored skin of adulthood, the elevated proportions of yellow, neutral xanthophyll esters diminish, while the totals of red, esterified astaxanthin and of orange 4-ketolutein increase.

Crozier conducted a comparative study on the carotenoids of seven local rockfish species belonging to the *Sebastes* genus. He correlated kinds and concentrations of carotenoids with general skin color. The investigations showed a range from vermilion down to olive-drab, through which astaxanthin decreased while neutral yellow xanthophylls, principally esters of tunaxanthin, increased, as shown in the accompanying chart.

Species	*Color*	*Carotenoids* (mg/100 g skin)	*Ratio of Esters*		
			Astaxanthin	Tunaxanthin	Zeaxanthin
Sebastes miniatus	Vermilion	7.5	76.8	11.6	11.6
S. constellatus	Orange	2.0	55.3	24.5	20.2
S. eos	Pale pink	4.5	47.5	33.8	19.3
S. umbrosus	Light orange	4.7	28.6	38.2	33.2
S. carnatus	Olive brown	1.2	22.9	60.5	16.6
S. flavidus	Gray-brown	4.9	20.1	46.7	33.2
S. atrovirens	Olive	1.9	0	87.6	12.4

AMPHIBIANS
(frogs, toads, salamanders)

As among fishes, the amphibian class includes species of bright yellow, orange, red, or combinations of such integumentary colors, once more due predominantly to carotenoids. The amphibians as a whole, however, are far less showy in coloration than are the fishes or the birds. They are, as a group, inclined toward drabness with notable exceptions, such as the strikingly pigmented fire-bellied toad *Bombinator igneus.*

The presence of carotenoids in general (or lipochromes as they were called in earlier years) was recognized in amphibians, as indeed in many other animal classes, in the last century. For example, they were identified in such species as the tree frog *Hyla arborea,* with its yellow skin, the common frog *Rana esculenta,* the toads *Bufo viridis, B. calamita, B. vulgaris,* and the orange-colored skin of the salamanders *Triton cristatus* and *Salamandra maculosa.* The ripe ovaries of *B. calamita* and adipose tissue of *T. cristatus* also yield such pigments. Even the blind and nearly colorless cavernicolous salamander *Proteus anguineus,* encountered in dark, underground caves of Italy and Yugoslavia, manages to obtain and store carotenoids from food transported by streams descending underground. Uncombined xanthophylls and β-carotene are present in *Proteus,* the former in the somatic tissues generally (minus the viscera), whereas the liver carotenoid is nearly all carotene.

The aforementioned familiar frog *R. esculenta* appears to have received perhaps the most searching study of its carotenoids as distributed in various tissues. This in turn reflects the fact that the species is relatively nonselective as to kinds of such dietary compounds, assimilating a wide variety.

Of its tissues analyzed, the fat-body was found to be richest in pigmentation, followed by the liver, ovaries, and skin, in that order. *Rana* tended, in general, to store roughly one-fourth to one-third of its tissue carotenoids as carotenes, while, of the xanthophyllic compounds, a ratio of about two to one prevailed, respecting esterified versus uncombined members, in liver, ovaries, and fat-body. However, in skin, a yield of some 1.36 mg per 100 g, the 25.4 percent figure for carotenes was augmented by 72 percent esterified, and only 2.6 percent free, xanthophylls; thus 96.5 percent of the stored xanthophylls were identified as esters, a condition imparting greater chemical stability.

Hugh Cott has described and illustrated a number of diurnally active but conspicuously colored amphibian species which, in view of their poisonous skin secretions, may thus enjoy a singular degree of immunity from attack by carnivorous predators. Some of Cott's exotic examples are the above-mentioned fire-bellied toad *Bombinator igneus,* the orange-and-black frog *Atelopes stelzneri,* the brilliantly crimson-marked frog *Phrynomerus bifasciatus,* the orange-yellow-black striped tree frog *Hyperolius marmoratus,* the fire salamander *Salamandra maculosa,* and the blue-spotted, pink-spotted, and orange-banded varieties of another frog, *Dendrobates tinctorius.* Cott points out that not all poisonous-skinned amphibians exhibit conspicuous integumentary pigmentation. A persistent question therefore lingers as to whether mucus-secreting and poison-secreting skins invariably require the presence of carotenoids. The substances in fact are known to be constituents of the mucus of some fishes, as well as the milky and waxy secretions of other animals. They are also known to be closely related

the A vitamins, which contribute to maintaining the moist surfaces of various tissues.

REPTILES
(snakes, lizards, turtles)

The skin colors of various snakes, lizards, and turtles are highly
diverse—often indeed striking and, among chameleons especially, changeable under control of nerve stimuli to the pigment
cells.

Notwithstanding, relatively little research has been devoted to
this vertebrate class. To be sure, studies even within the last century revealed alcohol-soluble pigments in the skins of a number
of snake and lizard species, but these pigments were not critically characterized.

The blood plasma of two Brazilian snakes, *Crotalus terrificus*
and *Xenodon merremii,* contain xanthophylls but no carotenes,
while two other species, *Bothrops jararaca* and *Eudryas bifossatus,* carry no carotenoid at all in their plasma, only small
amounts of a yellow, water-soluble, fluorescent flavin (see
flavins).

Chameleons depend upon four pigmentary or color-evoking
systems for effecting their striking integumentary chromatic
changes. These consist of dark melanins, within specialized,
branched cells; yellow carotenoids mainly in oil droplets and in
xanthophores; silvery or blue-scattering, platelike guanine crystals, stationary within so-called guanocytes or leucophores; and
an unidentified red material, all referring to an unnamed African species (see *Animal Biochromes*). The skin possesses a considerable quantity of xanthophylls (ca. 2 mg/100 g), about
three-quarters of which are esterified, and also traces of carotene. The ova yielded much free luteinlike xanthophyll, no
esters, and traces of carotene, while the liver was richest in total
carotenoids (ca. 10 mg/100 g), half of which, in one analysis,
were free xanthophylls, one-third were carotenes, and the
remaining sixth, xanthophyll esters.

The Florida chameleon *Anolis carolinensis* (L-G's "politico
lizard"), actually an iguanid type, carries a set of chromogenic

materials like those listed above for the African species, including yellow pigment dissolved in oil droplets and in special xanthophore cells—all readily extracted with alcohol—almost certainly carotenoid in nature.

Another distantly related species, the large, spiny-tailed iguana *Ctenosaura hemilopha* of southern North or Central America, bears a row of femoral pits or pores in the ventral skin of each thigh. These rounded, conical depressions in the male are filled with waxy kernels of a solid or semisolid secretion which can be squeezed out by manual pressure against the surrounding skin. That is, each funnel-shaped pore thus provides a waxy, yellowish or orange-colored cone which yields a yellow pigment to pure alcohol. The carotenoid found was a single, neutral, esterified xanthophyll doubtless acquired from the animal's vegetarian diet. The pigment's general chemical and spectral properties are closely reminiscent of taraxanthin, common in plants, or to tunaxanthin, found in the skin of marine fishes. Inasmuch as it has been derived from terrestrial plants, the compound is more likely allied to, if not identical with, taraxanthin, with a kindred spectrum.

The blood serum and stored fat of some tortoises are rich in carotenoids. In a few instances, turtle carotenoids have been characterized and classified. The red patch of skin near the eye of the small Japanese "painted turtle" has yielded a single, persistently carotenelike compound, spectrally resembling the red hydrocarbon γ-carotene encountered in certain species of dodder, among other plants. A yellow, carotenelike compound characterizes the yellow, upper surface of this turtle's shell. A yellow xanthophyll was found to accompany the same pigment in the viscera.

BIRDS

The avian class assuredly claims a superior position among all vertebrates, rivaling even the fishes in regard to variety and brilliance of coloration. There are, to be sure, many dull or cryptically colored species among the birds, and as to *skin* color, the fishes, and indeed some amphibians, truly excel. Among the

birds, while there are instances of bright facial and shank coloration, it is the feathers, which are lifeless, extruded, epidermal
material, that manifest the extraordinary displays of both pigmentation and structural coloration. Melanistic (black, brown,
and gray) and occasional porphyrinic colors share prominence
with the gaudy carotenoid plumage colors.

Lutein was the prominent xanthophyllic carotenoid first
recovered from egg yolks of domestic fowl, as well as from the
adipose tissue and integument of shanks and external ears.
Indeed, actively laying hens advertise their productivity by the
paleness of their legs and ears as the assimilated xanthophylls
are routed to the developing egg yolk instead of to other tissues,
which accordingly undergo a gradual loss of yellowness.

Cockerels display yellower legs, ears, and fat than do laying
pullets. The domestic fowl is a xanthophyll selector, assimilating only those carotenoids which possess at least one hydroxyl
radical on a terminal ring, and generally rejecting carotenes. It
would be interesting to know whether such birds assimilate such
ketones as echinenone and canthaxanthin, as do flamingos and
others. Hens fed a diet containing carotenes as the only carotenoid type have no difficulty in deriving therefrom their necessary stores of vitamin A, but otherwise store no more than the
merest traces of carotenoid—even to the extent of laying eggs
with colorless yolks, from which white chicks may hatch.

The yellow iris in chickens is carotenoid. (The red eyes of
pigeons, by contrast, owe their color to another kind of pigment.) Carotenoids indeed characterize the eye color of many
avaian species, including some Anseriformes (ducks, geese,
swans), Galliformes (grouse, pheasants, domestic fowl), Grui-
formes (cranes), Charadriiformes (gulls, auks), Strigiformes
(owls), Passeriformes (thrushes, warblers, etc.), and Ciconii-
formes (storks et al., including flamingos).

The Brazilian toucan *Rhmaphastos toco,* which feeds upon
plantains and other ripe or even rotting fruits, exhibits conspicuous red, orange, yellow, and black areas in the outer cuticle of
its huge bill, and bright red tail feathers. No carotenes are evident in either the bill cuticle or the red plumes. The cuticular
xanthophylls exhibit absorption maxima reminiscent of taraxanthin. No astaxanthin was identified. The feather xantho-

phylls differ from those of the bill, and include red, suspectedly more oxidized, fractions, but no recognizable astaxanthin.

Certain birds are able to alter dietary xanthophylls, such as lutein, zeaxanthin, and violaxanthin within the body, converting them into other xanthophylls. Zeaxanthin, for example, is converted by the canary *Serinus canaria canaria* from a yellow to a golden-yellow color, giving the new feathers an enriched hue with a red-orange tinge. Lutein feeding of this species resulted, however, in a bright-yellow feather color due to what was assigned the name "canary xanthophyll."

Like barnyard fowl, certain wild species such as the laughing gull *Larus ridibundus* and the stork *Ciconia ciconia* store no carotenes in their egg yolk. Nor do the yolks of these two birds yield luteinlike fractions, but rather chiefly a compound resembling astaxanthin. The difference is hardly surprising, in view of the two birds' subsistence mainly on aquatic animals. Even domestic fowl seem to store astaxanthin in the yolk when fed a diet including lobster or shrimp integument, and the same pigment finds its way into the retina of the unhatched chick.

The fulmar petrel *Fulmarus glacialis,* common in Arctic waters, stores considerable amounts of deep amber-colored oil in its proventriculus, or anterior stomach chamber. When disturbed upon its nest, this bird forcibly ejects through its gaping mouth quantities of this malodorous fluid; the oil functions also as food for its young. The carotenoids in the substance were found to be solely carotenes; no free or esterified xanthophylls nor acidogenic compounds such as astaxanthin were detected. It is not certain whether this carotenoid selectivity may reflect a strictly secretory source of the oil, which is rich in lipids and vitamins A and D or, alternatively, that it might be composed merely of undigested residual material. The former alternative would seem to be more likely.

Woodpeckers (flickers) and bishop birds or weaverbirds, as studied respectively by F. H. Test and H. Kritzler, afford examples of brightly colored feather patches (see *Animal Biochromes*). The flicker *Colaptes cafer* bears scarlet feathers, and *C. auratus,* yellow; an intermediate orange-colored form is believed to be a hybrid between the other two. This is not surprising considering the overlap of wild territories.

Yellow *C. auratus luteus* feathers owe their color principally to their storage of taraxanthinlike xanthophylls accompanied by minor amounts of a-carotene and some unknown red fractions.

The scarlet hues of *C. cafer* reflect the presence of red, spectrally single-maxima carotenoids. Moreover, yellow xanthophylls and orange carotenes accompanying the red fraction confer an orange tinge upon some feathers.

Flight feathers from the presumptive *cafer-auratus* hybrid are intermediately orange in color, and contain all three classes of carotenoid found in plumes of the two identified species, the red component of the hybrid's feathers constituting a smaller proportion of the total than in the case of *C. cafer*.

The display plumages of nuptially colored male bishop birds, *Euplectes,* are rich in several carotenoids, while the henny eclipse feathers, to which the males revert following the postnuptial molt, are nearly without such pigments.

From feathers of wild bishop birds *Euplectes franciscanus, E. orix,* and *E. nigroventris,* three carotenoids have been recovered: a red fraction, a yellow, luteinlike component, and a second red one showing spectral maxima different from the first compound. Captive *Euplectes* of all three species retained the first two carotenoids, but lost the second red fraction with the molt. Nevertheless, when fed capsanthin in the form of paprika, all three *Euplectes* species developed the latter carotenoid in regenerated feathers, as canaries have been known to do given this supplement.

More recent analyses and experimentation have provoked definite information regarding carotenoid metabolism in some birds. Working with the cedar waxwing *Bombycilla cedrorum,* Brush and Allen found astaxanthin to be solely responsible for the waxy red pigmentation conspicuously present at the tips of the nine secondary wing feathers. The pigment is found at the same site in mature individuals of both sexes, but not in all specimens, and never in the young.

Several species of *Rhamphocelus* tanagers from Central and South America show variations in the pigmentation of their rump feathers. The variation appears to occur among birds dwelling along a geographic, altitudinal cline. *R. flammingerus* from Colombia exhibits bright scarlet feathers, while *R. icteronotus,* ranging from Panama south to Venezuela, is characterized by a lemon-yellow hue instead, while *R. costaricensis* exhibits intermediate colors. The surprising development, however, is that all of the species, and various hybrids of them carry in the feathers but one and the same dihydroxyxanthophyll, resembling lutein or zeaxanthin, merely in different concentrations. Such a discovery suggests a persistently heritable, homeostatic kind of metabolic selectivity and assimilation, persisting through the several species of the one genus. This common metabolic property, and the fact of ready hybridization among the several forms, indeed prompts the inquiry as to whether all may not be subspecies or variants of a common species. Such questions must be left to be resolved by ornithological taxonomists.

With very substantial cooperative help from staff members and friends at the San Diego Zoo, it has been possible, over a number of years, to conduct, in the biochemical laboratories of the University of California's Scripps Institution of Oceanography, a considerable number of penetrating studies on the red ketocarotenoids characterizing the feathers, blood, and tissues of exotic wading birds of the tropics and semitropics. Such studies included work on the scarlet ibis, roseate spoonbill, and all six presently living species of flamingo. Some fifteen separate reports and about a dozen reviews, all issuing from this laboratory, have dealt with such work.

The roseate spoonbill *Ajaia ajaja* (pl. 10), resident in tropical and subtropical coastal regions of the southern United States to Patagonia, is a dabbler in shallow marshes and/or brackish waters, where it feeds on microscopic and other small organisms and much finely particulate detrital organic matter. The beautiful pink and deeper rosy shades of this bird's feathers reflect the presence of the two β-carotene-derived ketocarotenoids, canthaxanthin and astaxanthin, in that order of prominence. The pink tibiotarsal skin carries astaxanthin as the chief pigment. The same pigment is prominent also in the liver, in contrast with the condition in flamingos (see below).

The red-orange blood plasma from adult *Ajaia* contains about 1 mg carotenoid per 100 ml. The major pigment, comprising about three-fifths of the total, is canthaxanthin; another third is astaxanthin; a final small fraction of about 3 percent resembles phoenicopterone. Surprisingly, the former two fractions have been discovered also in the "ghosts," or empty membranes of laked red cells of the blood, but in concentrations amounting only to about one-fifth that in the plasma. The plasma carotenoids are firmly associated with lipoproteins.

The scarlet ibis *Guara* (formerly *Eudocimus*) *rubra* (pl. 11), another member of the heron family, shares with the spoonbill its tropical and subtropical habitats, subsisting upon generally similar kinds of food by digging into the sand, mud flats, or shallow bottoms with its long, slightly curved bill. Again, canthaxanthin is the chief carotenoid fraction in the red-orange plasma, red leg skin, liver, and brightly colored feathers.

No astaxanthin or other acidogenic carotenoid occurs in soft tissues, but feathers yield minor amounts of astaxanthin accompanied by a substantial fraction (ca. 13 percent of totals) of a new acidogenic carotenoid which we have called guaraxanthin, and which may be a dihydroastaxanthin derivative.

The liver, tarsal and toe skin, plasma and feathers of this bird are richer in carotenoids than are comparable parts of any other bird studied. Canthaxanthin is the principal carotenoid in all instances, ranging from 63 percent of plasma fractions to 90 percent of those in tarsal skin.

Researches by E. Trams suggest that the overturn time for plasma carotenoids in *Guara rubra* is relatively rapid. Their concentration falls away rapidly when the bird is maintained on a diet lacking such pigments. *Guara*'s span of but four days wherein the plasma carotenoids fall to half their original concentration is in contrast to what we have observed in flamingos; *Phoenicopterus ruber* plasma may not descend to the halfway level in carotenoid concentration until an elapse of some nine weeks. As in the roseate spoonbill, the ketocarotenoids in the plasma of this ibis are bonded with high-density lipoproteins.

The white ibis *Guara alba* carries in its plasma but minor amounts of recoverable carotenoids. The same is true of the Indian black-headed ibis *Threskiornis melanocephala,* which seems to store in its plasma none save faint traces of yellow pigment, and even in the liver there is only very little carotenoid, which is similar to canthaxanthin.

There occurs a pink-feathered ibis, apparently a hybrid from crossbreeding between *Guara rubra* and *G. alba*. Although apparently unable to transfer more than traces of carotenoid to its developing feathers, this suspected hybrid has been found to store in its blood plasma levels of carotenoid comparable with those found in *G. rubra* plasma.

Flamingos are the largest birds displaying major surfaces of bright red or pink feathers and exposed facial and tarsal skin. They derive this rich pigmentation and the deep orange-red color of the blood plasma from their metabolic capacity for oxidizing yellow or orange carotenes in their natural, largely plant, diet, to produce ketocarotenoids.

The six surviving species of flamingos are maintained in healthy flocks in the San Diego Zoo. They are:

American (Caribbean or West Indian): *Phoenicopterus ruber* (now *P. ruber ruber*) (pl. 10)
Greater or European: *Phoenicopterus antiquorum* (now *P. ruber roseus*)
Chilean: *Phoenicopterus chilensis*
Andean: *Phoenicoparrus andinus,* three-toed, with yellow shanks
James': *Phoenicoparrus jamesi,* three-toed, with red shanks
Lesser or Africa: *Phoeniconaias minor*

The generic name of each expresses the Greek equivalent of the birds' crimson color, for example, *Phoenicopterus:* crimson-winged; *Phoenicoparrus:* perhaps crimson bird of ill omen; and *Phoeniconaias:* crimson water nymph. The proposed interpretation of *Phoenicoparrus* would appear, however, to belie the prejudice endorsed by some Christian natives against killing the birds. When in flight aloft, with long neck extended and long legs aft, they look from below like crosses in the sky.

Despite the fact that flamingos consume in their finely particulate food substantial quantities of single-celled plant organisms and the remains thereof, and that these are preponderantly rich in neutral xanthophylls such as lutein, zeaxanthin, and other more plentiful, related members, the birds seem to store but little of such compounds. Nor do they seem capable of adding hydroxyl radicals to carotene molecules to generate xanthophylls. This is in spite of their hydroxylation of canthaxanthin (derived from β-carotene) to elaborate the hydroxyketo-carotenoids phoenicoxanthin and astaxanthin, stored ultimately in feathers and/or tarsal and facial skin. In fact, it seems that the two compounds are generated at the respective sites of deposition, not in the liver, where canthaxanthin is formed.

Based upon careful studies of the Caribbean flamingo, the most brightly colored of all six species, and also upon analyses involving feathers and tissues of the other five species, we have concluded that flamingos oxidize dietary carotenes, giving rise to the following five ketocarotenoid major products (the plus signs indicating relative prominence):

1. From β-carotene:
   Echinenone (4-keto-β-carotene; orange) in liver, blood, tarsal skin . . . . +
   Canthaxanthin (4,4'-diketo-β-carotene; red) in liver, blood, tarsal and facial skin, feathers, egg yolk . . . .
   . . . . + + + +
   Astaxanthin (4,4'-diketo-3,3'-dihydroxy-β-carotene; red) in feathers; and in tarsal skin of some species . . . . . .
   . . . . + + +
   Phoenicoxanthin (3-hydroxy-4,4'-diketo-β-carotene; red) in feathers; also in tarsal and facial skin of some species . . . . + +
2. From α-carotene:
   Phoenicopterone (4-keto-α-carotene; orange) in liver, plasma, skin; and traces in feathers of two species . . . . .
   . . . . +

Each of the above-listed carotenoid pigments of flamingo feathers and tissues was identified in the laboratory at La Jolla, although astaxanthin had been suspected in the fat of a flamingo as early as 1939 by Manunta.

There is in fact evidence for the assimilation of minor quantities of neutral, yellow xanthophylls derived from the plant food and carried by the blood to be deposited in the tarsal skin of Andean and James' flamingos. Indeed there is, in these two species a rare circumstance in that fucoxanthin (or perhaps fuco-

xanthinol), a chemically unstable but very prominent xanthophyll in phytoplankton and other marine algae, is stored in the
tarsal skin of both species. The condition is conspicuous in the
Andean bird, whose yellow legs attest to the storage of esterified fucoxanthinol and other xanthophylls in amounts aggregating about 22 percent of total carotenoids there deposited.
Much of the rest is canthaxanthin, the red color of which
occludes the minor proportions of fucoxanthinol and kindred
yellow xanthophylls in the tarsals of James' flamingo.

The yolk of a Caribbean flamingo's egg was found to be
fairly rich in carotenoids, the chief member present apparently
being canthaxanthin, accompanied by a minor echinenonelike
fraction. No astaxanthin was found, none being present even in
the blood of this species.

The milky secretion (crop milk) secreted from the crop epithelium of Caribbean flamingos, and used by the parents for
nourishing the nestling chicks, is of a bright red color, is of
nearly neutral pH (acid-base) level, and is nutritious in glucose
and fatty content. The red color reflects the substantial quantities of canthaxanthin present, accompanied by a little hydroxy-
xanthophyll and traces of β-carotene.

All six flamingos, like the roseate spoonbill and scarlet ibis,
store canthaxanthin as by far the prominent carotenoid in blood
plasma (pl. 12) and colored feathers.

Flamingos also store the red, related pigments astaxanthin
and phoenicoxanthin at secondary levels in their plumage. The
roseate spoonbill also bears astaxanthin in its feathers, in concentrations secondary to canthaxanthin. The scarlet ibis, storing but little astaxanthin proper with its feather canthaxanthin
seemingly replaces the former largely with guaraxanthin.

Astaxanthin and phoenicoxanthin occur rarely—even ques-
tionably—in flamingo blood plasma. Both are lacking in the
Caribbean bird; the Greater species carries a little of each; the
Chilean mere traces. Andean and James' flamingo blood yields
neither, while the African bird's blood exhibits traces of astaxanthin and minor amounts of phoenicoxanthin. As to the
shank skin, the Caribbean bird stores little or no canthaxanthin,
but, as with the Chilean, major concentrations of esterified
astaxanthin. The two montane species, *P. andinus* and *P.*

jamesi carry in their exposed skin both canthaxanthin and asta-xanthin; James' flamingo skin also includes a little each of phoenicoxanthin and echinenone. The African species has been reported by some European workers to bear in its red leg skin widely varying proportions of canthaxanthin and astaxanthin. However, we could detect none of the former pigment; 95 percent of the total emerged as esterified astaxanthin, the rest being phoenicoxanthin, mostly esterified.

The discovery of fucoxanthin (or fucoxanthinol, App., 13-14) esters in the leg skin of the Andean, and to a lesser extent in that of the James, as well as encountering a minor fraction of ϵ-carotene (along with β-carotene) in the liver of an Andean specimen recently captured in its native home, both clearly reflect these birds' consumption of planktonic algae as a considerable part of their natural diet.

Through controlled experimentation with a segregated trio of *Phoenicopterus ruber* in the San Diego Zoo, we demonstrated this species' ability to convert dietary β-carotene into its mono-ketone echinenone, and thence into the diketonic derivative can-thaxanthin; also noted was the oxidation of a-carotene to its monoketone phoenicopterone, named after its discovery and identification as a natural product in our laboratory. In either case, withholding the carotene from the birds' food led to a diminution of the ketones in their blood, while resumption of the carotene diet restored the blood levels of the derived ketones. We investigated also the possible utilization of several other individual carotenoids by adding each singly to the birds' diet for suitable periods of time. The results may be tabulated as shown on page 85.

It is virtually certain that the conversion of β- and a-carotenes into their respective ketones occurs in the liver, where such products are to be found abundantly. The formation of phoeni-coxanthin and astaxanthin, however, cannot be regarded as deriving from canthaxanthin at *that site,* they never having been found there or in the blood. The conclusion remains that these two red, hydroxyketocarotenoids are elaborated from cantha-xanthin at the respective sites of their ultimate deposition, that is, in exposed ectodermal and in feather-follicular tissues. The finding of these two compounds in minor or trace quantities in blood plasma of the European, Chilean, and African birds and of astaxanthin in the spoonbill's plasma would suggest that they must be formed, at least in some part, in the liver of those species.

Carotenoid	Assimilated	Metabolized	Products
β-Carotene	yes	yes	Echinenone, canthaxanthin
α-Carotene	yes	yes	Phoenicopterone
Lutein	very little	questionable	none in blood
Zeaxanthin	no	no	none in blood
γ-Carotene	no	no	none in blood
Lycopene	no	no	none in blood
Astaxanthin	early traces?	no	none in blood
Canthaxanthin	yes	yes	Phoenicoxanthin and astaxanthin in feathers and skin

MAMMALS

It is in this class of animals that we find very few instances of observable carotenoid pigmentation. Exposed mammalian skin owes its pinkish coloration to the hemoglobin in the subdermal capillaries, and its yellowish, tan, or darker colors to the presence of melanin pigments in epidermis, dermis, or both. Golden or even bright-red fur or hair exhibits the hues of various chemical stages of melanin, never carotenoids or porphyrins.

There are, to be sure, exceptions wherein the yellow color of carotenoids are perceptible in bare skin, as in the udder of certain cattle in some seasons, and in humans, notably children, who have been fed excessive amounts of carotene-rich foods, such as the pulp and juices of oranges, carrot root, yellow squash, and the like over long periods. The skin thus assumes a definite yellow pigmentation, as may even the sweat; the condition known as false jaundice, carotenemia, or xanthemia is not attributable to a disease and gradually disappears when excessive dietary carotenoids have been discontinued. An interesting feature concerning human carotenemia is in the clinically demonstrated role of dietary β-carotene as a protective agent against sunlight sensitivity in the blood-generated disease protoporphyria.

The pale yellow color of many mammalian blood plasmas, as well as in the deposits of fatty tissue, and even a similar pigmentation of nerves themselves, arise from the presence of carotenoids. Likewise the corpus luteum is rich in carotenoids which confer upon the organ the color from which its name was derived. The liver and adrenals also are particularly rich in carotenoids, although not visibly so as a general rule.

Unlike a number of invertebrate flesh-eating species, carnivorous mammals such as dogs, cats, and others, store very little carotenoid in their bodies, save in certain glands. Even certain omnivores, such as rats, are poor in these pigments. More arresting yet is the fact that even many typical plant-eating species, including sheep, goats, swine, and most breeds of rabbits, store no more than traces of these pigments from the rich supplies in their natural food. There exists, however, a strain of rabbits which constitutes an exception to the deposition of only *white* fats by this species (*Lepas cuniculus*). In that genetically recessive strain the adipose fat is of a bright orange-yellow color, exhibiting the presence of a xanthophyll. The pigmentation disappears if carotenoid-rich fodder is eliminated from the diet. The "yellow-fatted" genotype seems to lack an oxidative enzyme in the liver possessed by the dominant "white-fatted" strain, and responsible for the oxidative degeneration of the carotenoid.

Conditions among guinea pigs are closely similar to those applying to the dominant rabbit strain, in that blood, testes, spleen, and heart yield no carotenoids, and liver mere traces, while even the adrenals, usually a rich storehouse for mammalian carotenoids, yield only a fractional milligram of the pigment per 100 g. Experimentally fed carotene is not accumulated in any organ or fluid, but is discharged in the feces.

Certain larger mammals have been shown to store copious carotenoids in various sites. Whales, which consume vast numbers of small marine crustaceans, such as krill or euphausiids, have been found, as a consequence, to store much astaxanthin and traces of β-carotene in their stomach oil. Indeed, there have been reports of an occasional "red" specimen of blue whale, wherein the red carotenoid has been generally distributed into the body tissues instead of remaining mainly in the liver.

Much study has been given to the carotenoids of domestic animals, notably cattle and horses. The fat-soluble yellow pigments in plasma, corpus luteum, body fat, and notably in milk fat or butter have been recognized and discussed in publications dating back for nearly a century and a half.

Cattle blood plasma and butter fat are especially richly colored in the spring season while the animals are grazing on green grass. The yellow compound selectively stored by cattle is very largely β-carotene, although small amounts of the a-compound have been found, as well as lesser quantities of certain xanthophylls. These observations apply notably to butter.

Understandably, ovarian tissues are richer in carotene, by fourfold, than testes. And of the ovarian tissues the corpora lutea and corpora rubra are richest of all. The plasma of cows also exceeds that of bulls in carotene content, by three to five times. The liver and adrenal glands are also remarkably rich in carotene content. Oddly enough, carotene has been detected in the earwax of cattle and in the "yellow patch" of olfactory tissue near the upper end of the nasal cavity. In such carotene accumulators as cattle, it comes as no surprise to encounter substantial amounts of the pigments in the feces.

Carotene selectivity in cattle is emphasized by the fact that, although a-carotene is greatly subordinate in concentration to the β-isomer, or even completely lacking in some green grasses, it is assimilated to some extent by the consumers, whereas xanthophylls, which preponderate considerably over carotenes in green leaves and grasses consumed by cattle, are very sparingly assimilated.

Like swine, which store no carotenoids in blood plasma or

body fat, sheep and goats bear mere traces of the pigment at the same respective sites. This is true even when the animals are consuming fresh grass daily over several weeks' time.

The few specimens of antelope, deer, and buffalo which have been examined yielded but traces of carotene from their plasma or butter fat.

Like cattle, horses also accumulate considerable amounts of carotene from their mixed diet of plants. The horse, moreover, is completely selective of carotenes, assimilating no detectable traces of xanthophyllic derivatives in blood plasma, depot fat, liver, kidneys, adrenals, spleen, or lungs. Some 70 to 80 percent of ingested carotenes are rejected via the feces, and about 60 percent of the xanthophylls ingested reappear there likewise; the remainder of the latter doubtless are destroyed in the alimentary tract, whether by extracellular mucosal enzymes or endemic bacteria.

Unlike either the domestic fowl, which selects only xantho-phylls, the horse, which rejects these, assimilating only caro-tenes, or the pig, which excludes both kinds from its assimila-tion, humans are quite nonselective, assimilating both types equally readily, as do the lowly frog and octopus. The plasma usually carries rather minor quantities of carotenoids save under exceptional dietary conditions mentioned earlier, whereas the adult liver, spleen, and especially the adrenals and storage fat may act as relatively rich carotenoid depots in humans. Milk and colostrum may also carry fairly rich concentrations of these pigments.

The depot fat of human cadavers, as observed, for example, by students in human anatomy classes, may possess rich colors in countries such as Hungary, where much paprika and allied materials are eaten, thus affording unusual quantities of the red hydrocarbon lycopene (prominent also in tomatoes and water-melons), and the red paprika xanthophyll capsanthin.

DETRITUS AND SEDIMENT IN NATURAL WATERS

The carotenoids admittedly receive a major share of attention among colored biochemical compounds, not only because of their ubiquitous distribution among living plants and animals, their enormous total mass around the world (from an annual production conservatively estimated to be about 10^8 tons), and certain properties of vital importance, but because they are further distinguished by their surviving presence in nonliving matter of biological origin. We have considered examples of carotenoids in solid calcareous material in certain corals, in hard keratin-proteins and some feathers, insect wing covers, and so on, and in tough, chitinous crustacean armor. Not surprisingly, these pigments occur abundantly also in colloidal or other finely particulate organic matter, whether suspended as leptopel in oceanic or lake waters or associated with bottom sediments rich in organic matter, partly in thin carpets of so-called sapropel, and in greater part buried in organic-rich bottom mud, silt, or sand.

Phytoplankton, the richest source of organic matter in the world's waters, are photosynthetically active at levels receiving diurnal fractions of sunlight. And while countless swimming or sedentary animals derive their nutrition, and hence their carotenoid supplies, directly from the consumption of such plant cells, others acquire the same food elements indirectly. This may be a consequence of eating other animals or filtering and engulfing detrital, organic-rich residues suspended in deeper, dark waters, or scraping, sweeping or shoveling solid materials from ocean or lake floors into their digestive systems.

Carotenoids have long been identified in deeply buried marine muds, at depths exceeding 2,000 m from the water surface. Chlorophyll-degradation products are accompanied at such sites by algal carotenoids and others more characteristic of bacteria and fungi. Sediment cores from the Gulf of California, dating back about 7,000 years, and still older samples from Canadian lakes and pools, estimated at about 11,000 years since deposit, have yielded identifiable carotenoids.

Whereas in fresh plant cells the xanthophyllic compounds are far more prominent, amounting to as great as 90 percent of totals in some instances, it would appear that the carotene type outlasts the xanthophyllic fraction in long-buried sediments. Whether the reason for this may be chiefly a more ready degradation of the xanthophylls, or whether perhaps these substances are deoxygenated, reducing them chemically to carotenes by endemic anaerobic microorganisms is not known, but the latter has been suspected.

Certain it is, however, that the cold, lightless, oxygen-lacking environment provided by buried sedimentary organic materials must favor the stability even of relatively labile constituents such as the immured carotenoids.

This potential source of these colored molecules must contribute substantially to the supply of such pigments for various benthic, bottom-dwelling animals inhabiting the zone. These would include not only brittle stars, certain crustaceans, worms, and molluscs of the area, but deep-sea fishes and other animals of carnivorous habit, which may prey upon the mud-eating species, thus acquiring their carotenoids at secondhand or even less directly.

Passing mention should be made here to a water-insoluble, lipid-soluble, otherwise ill-defined class of pigments which simulate carotenoids in some superficial respects, and may be confused with them if accorded merely casual observation. These are the chromolipids, or lipofuscines, to use the older term. They are of rather wide occurrence among the lipids of animal tissues but hardly are important enough to merit a separate chapter in a survey of this kind. They are treated here chiefly because of their superficial likeness not only to carotenoids, on the one hand, but to melanins, on the other, when encountered by an inexperienced investigator examining animal materials.

The chromolipids exhibit yellowish, ruddy, brown, or blackish colors. Chemically, they are poorly defined oxidative derivatives of various lipid materials, prominently inclusive of long-chain fatty acids. Progressive oxidation is accompanied by a general deepening of color, often by increasing rancidity as acidic fragments of relatively reduced molecular size are disrupted from chromogenic residues. The process may be simulated through exposing pale fats to heating in the presence of atmospheric oxygen, a daily occurrence in the kitchen.

The chromolipids simulate carotenoids sometimes when one is trying to recover the latter pigments from a yellow animal material, and succeeds in obtaining a yellow (sometimes a rather "dirty-yellow") alcoholic extract. But, unlike carotenoids, these colored residues do not exhibit spectral absorption maxima bands in the blue or blue-green (and only sometimes in the far-violet) region. Unlike most carotenoids also, chromolipids may exhibit fluorescence when illuminated with ultraviolet light.

Further—now in contrast to melanins—the chromolipids contain no combined nitrogen. They differ also in the fact that, while dilute acids precipitate melanins, they do not affect chromolipids. Concentrated mineral acids such as sulfuric or hydrochloric, when added to carotenoid solutions, give rise to blue or green colors, which gradually fade; with chromolipids such acids produce an increasingly dark sludge. And there are other chemical distinctions which set this group of colored bodies apart from the other to which they bear superficial resemblance.

Chromolipids are particularly noticeable in brown or brownish depot fat, and in the adrenal cortex of dogs, cats, guinea pigs, horses, and aged humans. However, even fatty acids and their glyceryl esters, sterols and phospholipids, when merely stored in glass containers, exhibit gradual darkening with progressive atmospheric oxidation, a process which, as observed, is accelerated by heating.

In the animal organism, chromolipids may serve either as stores of fuel for the release of energy, as do other depot fats, or may play other important biochemical roles, such as serving as catalysts for oxidative metabolic processes. Indeed, brown lipid deposits contain cytochrome oxidase. In many ways, however, these pigmentary compounds resemble cumulative lipid wastes.

4

Quinones*

The quinone biochromes are best classified under four chief headings: a chromatically inconspicuous one, the benzoquinones, and three more commonly encountered types, the naphthoquinones, anthraquinones, and polycyclic quinones.

Benzoquinones find representation commonly in some fungi, in some roots, certain berries, as well as in galls (pathogenic growths) of higher plants, whence they are recoverable as yellow, orange, red, violet, or darker crystalline or other solid materials.

Minor quantities of pale-yellow crystals of one such representative, known as coenzyme Q, have been recovered as a pigment believed to be, or to closely resemble, a biochrome almost universally distributed in plants and animals. These Q-coenzymes are referred to also as ubiquinones owing to their nearly universal occurrence. The compounds are accorded only passing attention here, however, for they confer no recognizable pigmentation upon any organism, a result of their minute concentrations; but they do occupy a vital role as respiratory enzymes in accelerating intracellular oxidations (see the coenzyme Q_{10} member of the series, App. formula 31).

Naphthoquinones are discernible in many parts of higher plants, including leaves, seeds, roots, bark, and woody portions. They are found also in some bacteria, from which they are recoverable in yellow, orange, red, or purple crystals. They are soluble in organic solvents, and have been widely applied as dyes for fabrics.

Vitamin K, a phylloquinone, is a pale-yellow, viscous oil,

*Chemical formulas will be found in the Appendix, 31-37 and 42-46. See also pls. 6-9a, b.

recovered from green plants such as alfalfa and tomato, as well as from some microorganisms; it is applied medically to combat deficiency of prothrombin, the blood-clotting factor. Vitamin K_2, which combats hemorrhage, is recovered from certain bacterial species and from purified fish meal, in pale-yellow crystalline form (App., 35-36).

Naturalists have long recognized the principal members of this biochrome class as existing in the so-called echinochromes and spinochromes; they are polyhydroxynaphthoquinones and confer various red, purple, or brownish coloration on the shell, spines, skin, and internal tissues of sea urchins and sand dollars.

As with the carotenoids, however, the original synthesis of these quinones de novo seems to reside in plants, with few if any suspected exceptions. Moreover, despite their pronounced tinctorial properties as a class, only a few quinones are known to occur in appreciable quantities in animals. Indeed, animals known to store the naphthoquinones and anthraquinones in conspicuous amounts are limited to the above-named echinoid class, one holothurian or sea cucumber species, certain homopterous insects, and a few swimming crinoid species. There are, however, vertebrate marine animals which prey upon echinoids and adventitiously derive therefrom the naphthoquinone pigments, which they then deposit in their own skeletal parts. Examples include the sea otter, *Enhydria lutris,* whose purple and pink skeletal colors are derived from its heavy consumption of urchins, for example, *Strongylocentrotus drobachiensis.* A similar status applies to the dental and whole calcareous oral equipment and dorsal spine of the horned shark, *Heterodontus francisci* (pl. 9a, b) which consumes the same kind of prey. Indeed, purple-staining of the skeletons of young, growing mice was induced experimentally by V. Yadon, who fed the animals on (whole bodies of) finely ground, red sea urchins, *Strongylocentrotus franciscanus* (pl. 7) mixed with peanut butter as the chief ingredient.

It is the presence of the hydroxyl radicals within the condensed, aromatic ring structures of these compounds that renders them phenolic, thus mildly acidic in nature, and hence capable of forming salt complexes occurring in close association with the chief skeletal material of the organisms storing them with the calcium carbonate of echinoid tests and spines, and with calcium phosphate in the bones of the otter, horned shark, and experimental mice. The pigments therefore are recoverable by dissolving such skeletal materials in acidic media, best combined with a water-immiscible organic solvent such as diethyl ether, to dissolve the pigment as it is liberated.

Whereas spinochromes are characteristic components of the calcareous spines and test of an echinoid, the echinochromes, differing from the former only with reference to certain side chains (see App., 32-33), are found as well in soft tissues such as the elaeocytes or amebocytic cells of the coelomic fluid, eggs and egg jelly, ectodermal and endodermal tissues, including the gut, from all of which they may be recovered with a slightly acidified, water-miscible organic solvent, such as 80 percent acetone containing 1 percent acetic acid.

The echinochrome or spinochrome compounds are but slightly soluble in water or in hexane, but readily so in organic liquids of intermediate polarities, such as ether, acetone, or alcohol. Being mildly acidic, they afford water-soluble salts of sodium, or insoluble salts of calcium or lead.

These polydydroxynaphthoquinones are mildly oxidizing in that they may be chemically reduced, with discharge of their colors, by treatment with sodium hydrosulfite; the reaction is reversible, with ready return of the color, merely through shaking in air, or by treatment with any of several mild oxidizing agents. Like phenols in general, the free naphthoquinones exhibit green colors when treated with acidified ferric chloride.

These natural biochromes display clearly defined maximal absorption bands in the visible spectrum, important data in their diagnosis. Thus echinochrome A provides the following examples in four different solvents:

Solvent	*Absorption maxima*
Benzene	532, 494, 461 nm
Chloroform	533, 497, 462 nm
Carbon disulfide	535, 499, 464 nm
Conc. sulfuric acid	502, 469 nm

It is notable that the maxima, situated in the green, blue-green, and blue spectral regions exhibit but little difference in the three organic solvents, thus differing considerably from the spectral behavior of carotenoids. These naturally occurring quinone compounds are, moreover, present in higher concentrations in tissues than are the carotenoids, which occur usually in traces.

There are to date few clues bearing on any physiological function fulfilled by the naphthoquinone derivatives beyond the prothrombin or blood-clotting factor, Vitamin K_1 and the antihemorrhagic one K_2, both as applied to mammals (App., 35 and 36). As to the metabolic origin of these aromatic compounds, it would seem most likely that they, or in some instances colorless precursors of them, must be acquired from the echinoids' habit of feeding on plant materials. There remains, however, the puzzling observation of echinochromelike pigments within differentiating cells, even in the gastrula stage of embryonic *Lytechinus variegatus*. Similar observations have applied to two other sea urchins, *Strongylocentrotus purpuratus* and *S. franciscanus* (pl. 6-7). Echinochrome's appearance begins even prior to gastrulation in the former and, following this stage, in the latter species. A colorless precursor in the cytoplasm, derived originally from the parent's food, should be suspected and sought.

Not all echinoids store polyhydroxynaphthoquinones of the echinochrome and spinochrome type. Brief study has been given to two species in this respect, namely *Dendraster excentricus* (pl. 8) and *D. laevis,* respectively the purple and the light-brownish, so-called soft or smooth sand dollar (with short, relatively soft spines). The two species occur in neighboring, even contiguous or overlapping, sandy, underwater habitats near-shore in the San Diego area, where they are found to bury or partly bury themselves in slanting positions. The two species exhibit radical differences in their pigmentation, as well as in length and thickness of spines. *D. excentricus* carries aggregates of purple echinochrome in ectodermal and endodermal tissues lining the shell, in ripe gonads of both sexes, in foregut tissues, and in the gelatinous egg cases. With the application of dilute acid in appropriate organic solvents, the red echinochrome is extracted from tissues and shell.

The smooth urchin, *D. laevis,* yields no recognizable echino-chromolike material, but only a water-soluble, ether-insoluble green pigment. Preservation in dilute aqueous formaldehyde solution effected the leaching away from *D. excentricus* deep-port-wine-colored echinochrome, while *D. laevis* imparted to the same preservative only a conspicuous green color. Freshly collected *laevis* specimens may show green patches over the upper, external surface, where they may have been scraped, or where a barnacle may have once settled; indeed, when the deli-cate ectoderm is broken by rubbing or scratching, the same effects appear at once. Green pigment is released from such lesions into seawater or from the intact animal upon immersion into distilled water. The green pigment is reversibly rendered colorless by change of pH. Thus at levels of about pH 3 or below (e.g., in dilute acetic acid), the color is quenched, but returns at about pH 5, and the pigment is precipitated in murky green flocs at alkaline levels above pH 10. The raw aqueous solution shows absorption maxima at pH 5 as follows: 395, 436, ca. 516, and 620 nm, and at ca. pH 10, 395, 455, and 620 nm. The pigment is not chemically reduced, as in the case of the echinochromes and spinochromes, by hydrosulfite. Its identity remains unsolved, awaiting the compelling curiosity of some other comparative biochemist.

Echinochromelike compounds have been reported in other echinoderm species. The small, dark-purple holothurian *Poly-cheira rufescens* bears in its body wall such a compound, conju-gated with protein. In addition to this sea cucumber, another instance is the free-swimming crinoid *Antedon bifida,* which displays a colorless skeleton, but stores in its red ovarian and connective tissues a red polyhydroxynaphthoquinone.

No role of physiological significance has yet been recognized in echinoids for these biochromes. As a general rule, no mere biocatalyst, such as an enzyme, hormone, or vitamin, ever occurs in tissues at concentrations attained by these naphtho-quinone derivatives.

Anthraquinones (App., 37; 42-44) are brilliantly colored pig-ments of wide occurrence in plants, but again, incident in rela-tively few animal species, including representatives of certain insect groups and a limited number of free-swimming crinoid echinoderms, the only animals in the marine world yet known to store such pigments.

These phenolic anthraquinones have been widely applied as dyes for fabrics since ancient times. They are used also as chemical indicators for acidity or alkalinity.

Three of the best-known members of this group are carminic, kermesic, and laccaic acids, each of which has served as a brilliant red dye of commercial importance dating far back into antiquity.

Cochineal, the red potassium salt of carminic acid (App., 43) occurs plentifully in fat-body cells of the female scale insect *Dactylopius coccus,* which lives on the cactus *Nopalea coccinelifera* of Mexico and Central and South America. *D. ceylonicus* and other species store the same or a closely allied pigment. The cochineal is not limited exclusively to the adult fat-body, but is encountered also in the eggs, as well as in the fat-bodies of newly hatched larvae. The pigment may account for as much as 50 percent of the dry weight of the female insects' bodies, but occurs also, albeit in lesser proportions, in males, which reach only about half the size of their mates, and are outnumbered by them by as much as 200-fold. They also differ from the females in being winged, and without mouth parts, so they must have acquired their complement of the plant pigment at some earlier stage. While not found in the gut proper, the red compound has been identified in the insect's feces, perhaps arising from the tubules delivering near the end of the alimentary tract. The material is in all likelihood derived from the insect's plant food. No physiologically significant role has been assignable to the pigment.

Carminic acid, extracted from the dried insects' bodies in hot water which later is acidified, may be dissolved in ethanol, and therefrom crystallized by slow evaporation of the solvent, or by acidification of a strong aqueous solution with acetic acid. The crystalline compound shows no actual melting point but chars at 205°C. It displays characteristic absorption bands in several solvents, for example, in sulfuric acid at 544, 504, and 474 nm (see *Animal Biochromes*).

Kermesic acid (App., 42) a red dye widely employed in ancient Greece and Rome, is recovered from the female kermes

Lecanium ilicis, which thrives on many oak species in Portugal, Spain, and Morocco. Its hosts include the holm oak *Quercus ilex* and the evergreen alkermes oak *Q. coccifera.* The average yield of kermesic acid is about 1 percent of the raw material. Properties resemble those of carminic acid.

Lac dye, commonly accompanying shellac and other lacquer materials, is derived from several species of scale insects, including *Tachardia lacca,* abundant in India on such plants as *Zizyphus, Acacia,* and *Butea,* and from *Coccus laccae,* growing on many trees of the East Indies, Ceylon, and the Molucca Islands. The resinous material is secreted abundantly by the female insects, and constitutes, with the skin casts, a hard armor over their bodies. From this lac (derived from the Sanskrit *lakh,* denoting the number 100,000, suggesting the vast numbers of insects) is recovered the red, hydroxydicarboxylic anthraquinone compound laccaic acid whose chemical and physical properties, solubilities, and color all are generally characteristic of the previous two compounds.

Like their chemical relatives, the naphthoquinones, these anthraquinones also doubtless are derived by the insects from consuming parts of their plant hosts; yet we know at present nothing of their metabolism or possible physiological significance in either plant hosts or animal parasites.

Four relatively novel anthraquinone pigments, recognized in the marine world, all refer to such compounds encountered in certain free-living species of sea lilies or crinoid echinoderms, investigated by some Australian workers. The newly described compounds have been given names suggesting those of the species in which they were first encountered. Thus rhodocomatulin, a butyltetrahydroxyanthraquinone (App., 37), and rubrocomatulin, closely allied to it chemically, confer bright to dark-red or purple colors upon the ten-armed, swimming crinoids *Comatula pectinata* and *C. cratura,* whence they are extracted readily with acetone or similar organic solvents. From the purple "passion flower" *Ptilometra australis,* another free-swimming crinoid of the Australian coast, there were recovered a triplet of chemically allied, red trihydroxyanthraquinones, one of which is more acidic than the others in bearing a carboxyl radical. The latter compound was recovered also from both yellow and deep-purple specimens of yet another Australian crinoid, *Tropiometra afra.*

There are yet no clues as to the original sources of these poly-hydroxy, tricyclic quinones, stored by crinoid species even during the Jurassic period, dating back for 120 million to 155 million years.

It will be of some special interest, before leaving this rather tantalizing subject of the anthraquinones, to recall another instance of biochemical dyeing in vivo by such a compound. This refers to a purely adventitous event, resulting from the consumption of the red dye alizarin ($=$ 1,2-dihydroxy-9,10-anthraquinone, App., 34), a natural coloring material occurring in the red roots of such Madder plants as *Rubia tinctoria* and other *Rubia* species. Domestic cattle and other herbivorous animals fed over long periods on diets containing madder root acquire a conspicuous purplish-red pigmentation in the growing ends of their bones, from the calcification of the phenolic, hence mildly acidic, quinone, and its continuous deposition along with the skeletal calcium phosphate.

In ancient times, indeed, madder was long administered to, or voluntarily eaten by people for its believed medicinal value, and for its suspected role in warding off witchcraft. Mishnaic Jews (200 B.C.-A.D. 200) thus used it, and Middle Eastern Arabs reportedly attribute madder with magic properties, using it as a drink to forefend effects of the "evil eye." Man's consumption of madder in remote times is revealed by the discovery of alizarin as the purplish-red stain in human bones excavated from a 2,000-year burial in a cemetery at the ancient site of Qumran, Jordan, near the northwestern shores of the Dead Sea.

Polycyclic quinones, including *aphins* (App., 45-46) are relatively rare molecules occurring in certain bacterial and fungal species, and in parts of some higher plants. They are rare in animals, but compounds of the so-called aphin group derive this designation from their initial discovery in the circulating lymph fluid of a number of colored sucking lice or aphid species. These homopterous insects, like other quinone-assimilating species, parasitize plants. *Aphis fabae,* an example, feeds upon the sap of the broad bean plant *Vicia faba.* Other aphids having this basic habit are *Tuberolachmus, Myzus, Dactynotus,* and *Eriosoma,* which infest a large number of plant hosts.

The black aphid *Aphis fabae* has received some detailed study. If the fresh insects are leached with hot water they yield a water-soluble biochrome, protoaphin, recoverable as fine yellow needles.

Oxidative enzymes in the crushed insects convert protoaphin (App., 45) to a fat-soluble compound, xanthoaphin, which takes the form of small, bright-yellow needles when crystallized from carbon tetrachloride. Progressive oxidation converts this, in turn, to chrysoaphin, precipitable from the same solvent as orange-yellow microcrystals. This pigment, moreover, is further oxidized enzymically to erythroaphin (App., 46), crystallizable from chloroform and ethanol as deep-carmine-red needles.

Being endowed with hydroxy radicals at certain loci on their aromatic rings, thus in fact having a phenolic character, the aphins are mild acids. Yellow members of the group show pink or crimson colors on treatment with alkali, while erythroaphin, on similar treatment, changes from its clear-red color to a dark-green precipitate. The various aphin homologues display fluorescent colors when their solutions are illuminated with ultraviolet light.

Neutral chloroform solutions of three different aphins exhibit progressively longer spectral absorption maxima, as follows:

Xanthoaphin	433; 462 nm
Chrysoaphin	457; 488 nm
Erythroaphin	452 and 521 (both very faint); 564; 589 nm

These compounds have no characteristic melting points to aid us in their identification; they merely decompose while charring at temperatures beyond 300°C. Moreover, they cannot be sublimed from their solid state directly into vapor, even under high vacuum. They are readily soluble in pyridine, somewhat so in acetone, chloroform, or carbon tetrachloride, but sparingly in ethanol or ether. Being readily adsorbed on columns or thin layers of alumina, calcium hydroxide, or talc, they are easily resolved by chromatography.

No aphin molecule contains nitrogen, sulfur, or halogen atoms or methoxy radicals, but only carbon, hydrogen, and oxygen.

5
Flavonoids:
Anthocyans and Flavones*

In the flavonoids we find a class of nonnitrogenous, heterocyclic biochromes occurring widely in plants, but of very limited
incidence among animals; indeed they are confined to a few
insect and coelenterate species, which must derive the pigments
directly or indirectly from plant sources.

Flavonoids have a 15-carbon atom skeleton which is known
chemically as a 2-phenylbenzopyrone, bearing side groups of
hydroxyl or methoxy radicals. They occur naturally mainly as
glucosides, that is, condensed with simple sugar molecules.

Many compounds in this series, notably the anthoxanthins,
including flavones and flavonals, confer yellow colors particularly upon flower petals; the anthocyans also come under this
general class, and are water-soluble plant pigments of orange-
red, crimson, blue, violet, or other hues.

Of the anthoxanthin flavonoids, a prominent member is the
pale-yellow compound quercitin, isolated originally from an
oak genus *Quercus,* but of wide incidence among plant species.
When uncombined, quercitin is a weak acid, due to the presence
of several phenolic hydroxyl groups on the benzoid rings (see
App., 39). This anthoxanthin may often occur as a glycoside,
that is, having a hexose sugar, rhamnose, condensed with the
hydroxyl group in the 3-position. In this form it is known as
quercitrin, and possesses some interesting medicinal properties.
According to Varma and Kinoshita, the oral administration of
quercitrin to experimentally diabetic rodents, *Octodon degus,*

*Formulas will be found in the Appendix, 38-41.

decreases the incidence of cataract induced by the activity of an enzyme aldose reductase, which, as in galatosemia, brings about lens opacity. Quercitrin, it seems, inhibits the action of the enzyme, thus impeding the accumulation of sorbitol within the lens which otherwise would favor onset of the cataractous process.

Free quercitin itself, although a weak acid, unites with strong acids to give unstable orange salts, which dissociate readily in water. Quercitin can serve as a dye, yielding various colors according to the mordant used.

It hardly is surprising to come across flavones in tissues of insects which feed upon plant materials. Thus quercitin almost certainly is the pigment recoverable from the creamy-white to pale-yellow wing parts of *Melanargia galatea,* the "marbled white," an English satyrine butterfly whose wings become brilliant yellow in color when treated with alkalies or when exposed to gaseous ammonia. This color change is reversible. The butterfly reportedly derives its flavone pigment from feeding on *Dactylus glomerata,* or cocksfoot grass.

Flavones have been reported as occurring in certain hemipterous, sucking insects, or true bugs, suspectedly also in silkworms, as well as in some butterflies. Bugs found to contain flavones were characteristically parasitic upon plant juices, but one, the Philippine assassin bug *Eulyes illustris,* derives its flavone material by preying upon plant-parasitizing insects.

Flavonoids are believed to fulfill in some instances a physiological role recalling that of vitamin P. As an instance rutin (= quercitrin, already cited as an anticataractous agent) is believed to accelerate restorative processes subsequent to severe X-ray damage, and to prevent capillary fragility.

Payne, in 1931, reported that some hydroid coelenterates contain carotenoids but lack flavonoid pigments, while others exhibit the reverse condition. Five such latter hydroids, storing flavonoid pigments, were *Thiuaria articulata* (orange-brown), *Sertularia argentea* (white, but yellow in ammonia), *S. gayi* and *S. polyzonias* (both yellow), and a brown species, *S. pumila.* All pigment extracts showed yellow or brown coloration in mild alkali, but were colorless in dilute acid solution. All yielded colored salts of lead and ferric and ferrous iron. It is not easy to surmise the possible source of such typical plant pigments occurring, as these did, in carnivorous marine animals. For whereas carotenoids indeed abound in marine algae, flavones are not so reported.

Claims have been made that some flavonoid pigments, whether administered by mouth or by injection, appear in mammalian urine, while others are metabolically degraded. Again, these compounds, common in many plants, are of fortuitous manifestation in animals, where their physiological importance is questionable, save in the instances cited above for quercetrin.

Flavonoid glycosides, including those of quercitin, luteolin, and apigenin, have been encountered, along with phaeophorbide *a* from the corresponding chlorophyll compound, and other organic biochemical residues, in greenish, fossilized leaves of the elm family, such as *Celtis* and *Ulmus* genera. The integrity of such compounds, after periods of fossilization dating back for 25 to 36 million years, serves usefully in geochronological calculations, and indicates that the particular specimens must not have been exposed to environmental temperatures exceeding about 80°C nor to pH levels far from neutrality, or beyond the range between 6.3 and 7.2 during the postdepositional period.*   The anthocyans, including the uncombined, so-called anthocyanidines and their glycosides, the anthocyanins, are high-melting, large-molecular, crystallizable 2-phenylbenzopyrilium salts, bearing one or more hydroxyl groups on each ring. They differ from the closely related flavones only in not bearing a ketone group (App., 38-41).

We see and enjoy daily evidence of representative anthocyan compounds when contemplating the appeal of red, violet, or blue colors and patterns in many blossoms, fruits, leaves, or other plant tissues, where these compounds occur in cell sap. In some petals, anthocyans may account for high proportions of the total dry weight, up to 20 percent in some red dahlias, and even 33 percent in dark-blue pansies. The color of *Hydrangea* and other blossoms may be changed gradually from blue to pink, as does litmus paper in the laboratory, merely by rendering the soil slightly acidic, for example, with iron salts; the

---

*These findings were reported in *Science* by Giannasi and Niklas in 1977.

change is made reversible by mixing ashes with the soil. Conversely, red slices of beetroot assume a reversible purplish-blue color in vinegar, doubtless from the presence of a natural indicator which behaves in a manner opposite to that of litmus, and more like the response shown by Congo Red dye.

While these aqueous-soluble anthocyans commonly are recovered as their chlorides in the laboratory, they usually occur combined with natural organic acids in plants. They are not soluble in ether, chloroform, or benzene, but dissolve to some extent in water-miscible solvents such as alcohols.

Intense light and low winter temperatures induce development of anthocyanins, which replace the decomposing chlorophyll. These pigments may also serve as indicators of nutritional mineral deficiencies in plants. Shortages in the availability of phosphorus, potassium, magnesium, or boron are particularly so advertised by plants. Thus, leaves and stalks of certain types of corn develop purple colors during a lack of soil phosphate, while the appearance of brown, bronze, purple or red patches in leaves often signals potassium lack in soils supporting the growth of potato, cotton, cabbage, apple, and orange.

Lack of boron induces a red pigmentation in certain clover and alfalfa leaves, and insufficiency of magnesium leads to a development of cotton leaves colored a striking purplish-red between the dark-green veins. The genesis of anthocyanins in response to such nutritional deficiencies is not universal, but can occur only in those plant species endowed with genetic factors required for the biochemical synthesis of such pigments.

A typical anthocyanin exhibits red color in acidic media, blue in alkaline, and violet in neutral systems. Thus, while the same anthocyanin is expressed in blossoms of the blue cornflower, the red cornflower, red rose, and deep-red dahlia, the differences in color are evoked by corresponding variations in relative pH, or acid-alkali balance, of the natural cell sap.

There exist three chief, basic anthocyanidins in plants. These are cyanidin, pelargonidin, and delphinidin, all three of which have the same molecular architecture (App., 40 and 41).

During fruit canning, liberated anthocyanidins may form relatively insoluble salts with tin and iron, following attack upon the can metal by natural fruit acids. Thus corrosion rate may be accelerated by the initial presence of anthocyanins in high concentrations, resulting in a depression of quality and marketability.

Anthocyans appear in few animal species, all of those being insects. Larvae of a beetle. *Cionus olens,* carry water-soluble anthocyan material colored blue-violet or orange, according to prevailing pH conditions. The larva of a hymenopteran, *Athalia spinarum,* may carry a blue pigment, while a red-brown is observed in the robber fly *Asilus chrysitis.* In an aphid species, *Tritogenaphis rudbeckiae,* a vermilion-colored anthocyan was reported, and certain red anthocyans have been suspected in migratory locusts.

It is generally believed that the fortuitous acquisition of anthocyans by certain herbivorous insects, or by others which prey upon such species, serves no physiological advantage in the animal's metabolism, nor does the accumulation appear to be harmful.

6
Indole Pigments: Indigoids and Melanins

With this chapter we begin the review of naturally colored molecules involving the additional element nitrogen, bonded to certain carbon atoms in so-called heterocyclic ring formations. We shall consider three classes of endogenous biochromes involving combined nitrogen. Of these, the indigoids arise from metabolic degradation of the amino acid tryptophan, while the largest and by far the most widely occurring class, the melanin group, originate from the progressive oxidative degradation of another, equally important amino acid, tyrosine, and the polymerization of the products generated in the process. A third type, included here because of its imitation of melanins in some respects, belongs to the so-called ommochromes, classed chemically as phenoxazones. They are generated through the breakdown of tryptophan—as indeed are the indigo pigments—but they are of a different, more complex structure compared with the latter.

INDIGOIDS
(App., 47-51)

The commonest members of this class of compounds are the colorless molecules, indole and its 3-methyl derivative skatole, both generated during the putrefactive decomposition of tryptophan (in protein materials) by endemic intestinal bacteria. These compounds are mildly toxic and undergo detoxifying oxidation in the body, whether in the gut itself or after absorption therefrom into the blood; they give rise respectively to indoxyl and skatoxyl. Further detoxication involves conjugation with sulfuric acid, with accompanying conversion to the corresponding potassium salts. Further oxidation, followed by coupling or polymerization yields indigoid and melanoid biochromes (App., 52).

Free indole and skatole are expelled in feces, while indoxyl and skatoxyl salts—mainly potassium indoxyl sulfate (indican) —are excreted in the urine of various animals, notably in that of herbivores such as horses and cattle, as well as in cases of human liver cancer.

Indican, when present, is readily demonstrable in urine or other biological fluids by applying mild oxidizing agents such as potassium chlorate or ferric chloride to an acidified sample, then shaking with a few drops of chloroform, which then extracts the blue oxidation product indigo.

Under unusual circumstances, minute granules of indigo pigment may be discovered by microscopic examination of pathological urine samples. Indigo red (indirubin or indipupurin) is encountered on occasion in such urines as an isomer of indigotin (indigo blue), and arises in a similar manner from the action of infective bacteria.

Indigoid pigmentation may appear in voided urine merely on its standing, due to bacterial putrefaction. But the manifestation of blue or red pigmentation in a freshly voided urine specimen (indigouria) usually indicates bacterial infection within the bladder. Indigo pigments have been identified in kidney stones, bladder stones, ovarian cyst fluid, and even in perspiration.

Indigotin itself (App., 47) is recoverable as a deep-blue crystalline substance with a coppery-red, metallic glance, and melts at 390-393°C with decomposition. The crystals may be sublimed as a fiery red, violet-tinged vapor, which solidifies on a cool surface in rhombic crystalline form. Indigotin is insoluble in water, ether, and dilute acids and alkalies; it dissolves with difficulty in cold ethanol, more readily when warmed; and it is soluble in boiling aniline, in chloroform, boiling turpentine, paraffin, petroleum, and vegetable oils. A fine aqueous suspension of the pigment affords a poorly defined absorption band in the red spectral region, but more definite maxima are manifested in organic solvents such as benzene (purplish-blue solution: 599 nm), chloroform (blue: 601 nm), or aniline (green: 630 nm).*

The indigoid biochromes are not conspicuous in tissues of humans or other mammals, but are commonly of excretory incidence or of pathological significance. It may be recalled, however, that man has long applied indigo as a blue, body-decorating pigment. The ancient Britons used, in Caesar's day, to crush masses of the cruciferous plant *Isatis tinctoria,* then called "weld" or "woad," found growing around chalk pits and other sites of the English countryside. The resulting fermented paste thus obtained yielded the blue pigment, indigotin, which the natives smeared over their faces and bodies, partly perhaps as a mere decoration, but intended also to strike fear into invading enemies.

Biochromes of the indigo class are of minor and incidental occurrence among man and other mammals, and indeed in animals generally, although there remain examples, including the arresting and long-known purple secretion of certain marine snails in the *Murex, Mitra,* and *Purpura* genera. This so-called Tyrian Purple, or Purple of the Ancients, is 6,6'-dibromindigo (App., 51), the pigmentary secretion from several species of the named genera. It is believed, indeed, to have been the dye marketed by "Lydia, a seller of purple, of the city of Thyatira" (Acts 16:14), an early convert of the apostle Paul. The pigment originates as a precursor in the so-called purpurigenous gland, a strip of pale-yellow tissue overlying the rectal segment of the snail's gut, and known therefore as the adrectal gland. Because of its site beneath the animal's gill, it is known alternatively as the hypobranchial gland.

The separated purpurigenous glands from specimens of *Murex brandaris,* or of kindred marine snail species similarly equipped, may be spread upon paper and exposed to air and light. This gradually evokes the enzymic oxidative generation of the pigment, which is recoverable after the mass has been macerated in dilute sulfuric acid, washed and extracted with hot water and ethanol, and leached out finally in warm, water-

*Analogous properties of the less common isomer indirubin (App., 48) are reviewed also in *Animal Biochromes,* 2d ed., pp. 217-218.

immiscible organic solvents, such as tetrachlorethane or ethyl benzoate. Glittering, copper-colored microcrystals of the dibromindigo appear as the system is allowed to cool.

Dibromindigo is insoluble in water, cold ethanol, ether, or in dilute aqueous acids and alkalies; it dissolves to give red to redviolet solutions in numerous organic solvents, notably when heated.

In warm tetrachlorethane the compound manifests a broad absorption maximum in the orange region, centering at ca. 596 nm. In greatly attenuated solution the locus of the band appears in the yellow-orange, with its midpoint close to 585 nm.

We do not yet know whether the gastropod species storing the purple indigoid pigment actually brominate it in their metabolism. Nor has a physiological role of any kind been assigned to it. Despite its confinement to the cells of a specialized gland (as the colorless precursor), the compound has to be regarded, at least provisionally in view of its catabolic character, as more of an excretory waste product. Such an interpretation is emphasized by the occurrence of some indigoid pigments in the organic matter of the shell.

MELANINS*

By virtue of their nearly universal distribution and wide incidence in living species, these compounds constitute by far the major biochromes in this class. Indeed, they rival even the carotenoids in their near universality of conspicuous occurrence in animals (pls. 33-37), although by no means so in plants. Unlike the carotenoids, synthesized de novo only in plants, the melanins are endogenous in animals' metabolism, and indeed in some plants. Their black, gray, brown, tawny, or buff colors are manifest in many feathers, in hair, wool, fur, eyes, and skin of mammals, including man; in scales and integument, or both, of many species of fish, amphibians, and reptiles; in the secreted ink of octopus, squid, and a few fishes; and in the skin and various other tissues of many invertebrate animals. Black melanin

*App., 52; pls. 33-37.

pigment is observable also in some black skin moles of humans (*black* ones, not brown, usually are removed surgically), and notably in certain tumors (melanomata) of humans and other mammals, domestic fowl, axolotls and other amphibian forms, numerous reptilian species, and many fishes. Such tumors belong to the reputedly most malignant and rapidly growing cancerous types; thus they can be dangerous unless dealt with surgically or in alternative ways at an early period in their development.

Melanins are readily generated in fluids and tissues of some higher plants, examples being encountered in the cut surfaces of apples or potato tubers, which quickly redden and deepen further, even to blackness in the latter with lengthening exposure to air. The same is true of certain stem saps, an example of which is encountered in the "poison oak," *Rhus diversiloba,* native to the western United States. When a green branch or twig of this plant is broken, the poisonous sap may ooze out onto the hand of an unwary person, and there blacken very quickly, thus affording a visible warning to wash the part quickly. The affected skin is then commonly treated with a freshly prepared alcoholic solution of iron (*ferric*) chloride in order to oxidize and thus detoxicate the poisonous triphenolic compound lobinol, which otherwise evokes severe reddening, itching, and spreading dermatitis in most persons. Certain alternative oxidizing agents may be used in place of ferric chloride; the latter does, however, remain in solution, not being reduced to the ferrous state too quickly by the alcohol, which aids greatly in conducting the iron salt into the skin. Moreover, ferric salts are specifically useful in the ready oxidation of phenolic compounds.

Melanin pigments are encountered also in certain black, yeast-like torulas, fungi with brown or black hyphae, fungal spores, and black species of bacteria such as *Bacillus niger.*

Many animal tissues give evidence of possessing tyrosinase, though not always expressed by generation of melanin in situ. An example is the matte-white, or even the red, color variant of the plumose sea anemone *Metridium senile.* If the tissues of this animal be ground or minced and left exposed to air, the black pigmentation of melanin can be observed, progressing slowly from the surface downward into the body of the tissue-brei.

Other animals, including certain varieties of the above species, generate limited amounts of dark malenins in various parts of their bodies.

Chemical Properties

No melanin is a single, so-called stoichiometric compound, i.e., with a definite, reproducible molecular structure and weight. Rather, the melanins are amorphous, polymerized complexes generated typically by the progressive oxidative degradation of simpler molecules, principally the nearly ubiquitous amino acid tyrosine, a process catalyzed during certain steps by the copper-containing enzyme tyrosinase (scheme shown in App., 52), or related phenolic compounds such as p-cresol, p-aminophenol, tyramine, and other kindred compounds, including phenol itself. Bacteria may thus convert any of a number of such compounds into melanins, whereas the most common metabolic precursor of such pigments within an animal's body normally is tyrosine, a component of most proteins.

Melanins are extractable from hair, feathers, wool, or scales with hot, very dilute alkali, from which they finally are precipitable by mildly acidifying the system. The pigment material then recoverable by centrifugation or filtration appears as a jet-black, granular mass which may be dried to yield a very dark brown powder. Undried melanin usually may display immediate solubility in alkalies, dilute formic acid, dilute or glacial acetic acid, sodium monohydrogen phosphate solution, or even in very dilute mineral acids. From acidic or alkaline solutions, half-saturated ammonium sulfate or 1 percent hydrochloric acid effect ready precipitation.

If dried with the aid of heat, melanin alters its character to some degree in that it becomes insoluble in all the above solvents save alkalies, to which it now yields slowly and incompletely. However, if allowed to dry at moderate room temperatures, the melanin residue can be dissolved slowly but completely in dilute HC1 solution.

Heating dried melanin powder produces fusion at high temperatures, with decomposition, however, and the release of pyrrole and other organic nitrogen compounds.

An ash-free preparation of melanin from black sheep's wool was found by R. A. Gortner to show the following chemical components, in respective percentages: C: 52.6; H: 7.28; N: 13.42; S: 1.33, and O (by difference): 25.37. Such values correspond to ratios expressed by Gortner's original empirical formula: $C_{105}H_{173}N_{23}SO_{38}$.

Treatment with alkalies, save in very dilute concentrations of about 0.2 percent or less, and at mild temperatures, extensively modifies the chemical makeup and solubility behavior of melanin material. Thus strong concentrations of sodium hydroxide have been observed to effect a decrease in the nitrogen and hydrogen ratios, with a rise in proportions of carbon and oxygen, while the sulfur content seemed (surprisingly) to remain nearly unmodified in its proportion. Since sulfur, in its reduced state, such as in sulfide, is rather easily detached by alkaline treatment of an organic compound, this observed relative constancy in its proportional presence may conceivably have been one result of the partial chemical decomposition of the overall substance. The ability of melanins to dissolve in alkaline media, giving colloidal sols at any rate, doubtless derives from the presence of mildly acidic, terminal carboxyl and phenolic radicals in the polymerized material.

Melanins may be dissolved in concentrated sulfuric but not hydrochloric acid. Dilution of such a sulfuric acid solution of the pigment precipitates the material, but very likely in a somewhat altered chemical form, since this acid is a drastic reagent and, at high concentrations, can perform an oxidizing function. Some melanins can be dissolved in organic liquids, such as diethylamine or ethylene chlorhydrin. They are oxidatively bleached by such reagents as hydrogen peroxide, chlorine, bromine, chloric or chromic acids, or potassium permanganate. A diagnostic histochemical test for melanins is based on their capacity to reduce ammoniacal silver ions to black, metallic, powdery silver.

Melanin pigment proper often is quite black, or very deep brown in situ, while melanoproteins (wherein the polymer is chemically conjugated with protein material) commonly are of tan or other light-brown colors, as in some human skins and in the ink of the squid *Sepia officinalis,* and probably in the case of other cephalopods which eject brown ink. Similar ink is present as well in specialized glands of a few fish species, such as the crestfish *Lophotus* which, when alarmed, responds like the octopus with a vigorous expulsion of black pigment through a postanal vent due to muscular contractions against the two branches of the gas bladder resting against respective sides of the ink sac.

The presence of certain other oxidative enzyme-and-substrate systems, or of particular chemical compounds, in tissues, may regulate or even obstruct and preclude the enzymic oxidation of tyrosine, ordinarily leading to melanogenesis. Oxidases such as the one responsible for catalyzing the oxidation of the purine compound xanthine, or another such biocatalyst implementing the oxidation of the labile compound ascorbic acid (the anti-scurvy vitamin C), are good examples. In the presence of such systems, melanogenesis is precluded, whether in vivo or in laboratory vessels. Fresh human epidermis (but not the corium or dermal layer below) has been shown to contain water-soluble compounds bearing sulfhydryl (-SH) radicals, e.g., glutathione, which, perhaps through their more ready oxidizability, inhibit the enzymatic generation of melanin. It has been suggested that melanogenic stimuli, such as protracted exposure to sunlight, X rays, or heat, or the incidence of certain inflammatory diseases, may lead to the oxidation of the inhibitory -SH compounds, thus opening the way for the enzymatic reaction which fosters melanin formation. Physiological advantages attributed to melanins are (1) increased screening against injurious light rays, notably in the shorter wavelengths; (2) accelerated rates of heat exchange, whether by absorption or radiation; (3) enhanced toughness and mechanical resistance, through a kind of "tanning" of the hard protein; (4) diminished wettability, and (5) defense against desiccation.

The silky cock, endowed with white feathers but black integument, mesenteries, pia mater, and intermuscular connective tissues, contributes the melanistic pattern only to his daughters, by a melanin-free hen. Silky fowl wattles are deep purple as a consequence of the red color of hemoglobin superimposed upon Tyndall-blue scattering colors, emphasized by the underlying melanin deposits.

Careful experimentation in many laboratories has demonstrated that dark-colored substrates, or darkish backgrounds in general, favor the increased elaboration of melanophores, or melanin-containing cells, in the skin of some amphibians and in many species of marine and freshwater fish. The axolotl salamander *Ambystoma mexicana,* the frog *Rana temporaria,* and such fishes as the Pacific killifish *Fundulus parvipinnis* and the long-jawed goby *Gillichthys mirabilis,* both marine, and freshwater species such as the guppy *Lebistes reticulatus* and mosquito fish *Gambusia patruelis* are all examples. They were investigated by F. B. Sumner and shown to possess this capacity to synthesize more melanin and to elaborate more melanophores to carry it when exposed to light from above dark-bottomed, dark-sided aquaria. Moreover, the greenfish or opal-eye, *Girella nigricans,* for one example, not only undergoes—on dark backgrounds—increases of its integumentary melanin, but also diminution of white or silvery guanine within its so-called leucophores. These two biochemical effects may be reversed when the animals are kept in all-white surroundings, thus establishing extraordinary biochemical alterations in the metabolism of both tyrosine and the purine guanine as a consequence merely of the overall incident illumination entering the eyes. The subject needs further biochemical study.

Fishes in a lighted environment, but deprived of sight in both eyes whether by masking or by surgical enucleation, deposit somewhat increased amounts of integumentary melanin, thus appearing gradually darker in hue. Sighted fishes or amphibians, by contrast, maintained in total darkness undergo paling, with decreased skin melanin.

Classical experiments by Sumner clearly showed that fishes indeed profit by so-called protective coloration due to their disposition of skin pigment. *Gambusia* mosquito fishes induced to become black by long residence within blackened tanks, lighted from above, suffered far less from predation than did their contrasting, pale counterparts, newly transferred from all-whitened aquariums to the same dark tank with the resident population, when exposed to attack by such predatory birds as night herons or penguins, or by carnivorous sunfish. And the relative proportions of casualities were reversed when the darkened and paled phenotypes were exposed together, this time in the whitened tanks, in which the darkened fishes were very conspicuous to both observer and predator. The capacity of such animals to match somewhat the shade of their surroundings confers upon them a corresponding facility of escape from ready detection by a searching enemy.

The very minute micellae of melanoproteins lie within the colloidal range of size, that is, from 1 to 100 mμ (1 μ being about 1/25400 in.), and thus invisible in the compound microscope, whereas melanin particles themselves take the form of minute ellipsoids of ca. 0.30 to 0.45μ in major axis, and some 0.25 to 0.40 μ in minor axis; or they may be spherical, or nearly so, with diameters of 0.30 to 2.00 μ. Samples of dark human skin have yielded rodlets (0.1 $\times$ 0.4 μ to 0.18 $\times$ 0.60 μ) and spherules of 0.20 to 0.30 μ in diameter. They thus lie within the discernible size range of high microscopic powers.

Melanogenesis is induced by protracted exposure of the human skin to direct sunlight, thus promoting "tanning," practiced particularly in the southwestern United States, reportedly is accompanied by higher incidence of skin cancer. Tanning appears to be under some endocrine regulation. Castration, for example, is known to lead to mere burning and inflammation instead of tanning. If the male sex hormone testosterone is injected some days after exposure to the sun's rays, however, melanogenesis may be achieved in various tissues.

The structure of pelages, both hair and fur, of many mammalian species has received much study. Human hairs involve a cortex bearing cylindrical scales externally, surrounding the central medullary column or pith. These fluid-filled, so-called fusi extend upward as the hair shaft lengthens until no fluid remains, leaving the vessels compressed as delicate, lengthy, dark strands. Most of a hair shaft is constituted of multiple solid, partly translucent, elongated, and closely packed cortical cells, within which are scattered minute, roundish melanin bodies, giving the cortical column a pale-buff, brownish, darker, even black color depending on relative numbers and color depth of individual particles. Some animals' pelages bear melanin within the medulla or pith itself. The cortical melanin may occur as a colloidally dispersed brown stain, that is, as a melanoprotein, rather than being distributed in microscopically discernible particles.

Light-blond hair involves minor quantities of pale melanin material, whereas human red hair carries an iron-rich pigment recoverable, when dried, as an amorphous dark-red-brown powder, insoluble in acetic acid, but soluble in alkali. It is thus in some ways reminiscent of the melanins, and probably coexists with melanins in grades of ruddy, auburn, or russet-colored hair.

White hair or fur, for example, of albinos or polar mammals, contains pithy columns of air-filled, solid froth in place of the diffuse melanin pigment. Earlier the comparably sizable bubblets of air in alveolar cells of feathers as the responsible agency evoking the whiteness of total light-scattering was considered.

Populations of several species of moth or kindred lepidopteran forms are modified by adaptive so-called industrial melanism. One such instance is the British peppered moth *Biston betularia,* which occurs in two genotypic color phases, namely a light, variegated or "peppered" type and a melanistic variant. The light-colored or peppered type enjoys a considerable degree of concealment while resting on the color-matching surfaces of dry lichen covering the local oaks of the countryside, while the black specimens alighting there are most conspicuous, and thus readily seen and eaten by birds.

Conversely, the killing of the lichens by soot, which blackened the oak trunks in industrial sites, afforded a high degree of chromatic concealment to the black-colored *Biston* variant alighting thereupon, while their pale-toned kin resting at the same site thus proclaimed themselves to be prey.

The circumstance led to a noteworthy contrast between color types prevailing in communities occupied by the insect. The sooty industrial environment accommodated populations of nearly all-black specimens, whereas the country dwellers were predominantly of the pale-colored phase. Ultimately, pursuant to the enactment of laws against excessive burning of soot-generating fuels and the cleaning of sooty surfaces of trees and other perpendicular structures in industrial areas, reports were received of the reappearance of the lightly tinted *Bistons* in such cities. The moths could now again discover pale, matching substrates, and thus, through the camouflage afforded, return their earlier genotypic ratios to the local populations.

Melanistic blackening of predatory, deep-sea fishes' bodies serves readily to conceal them from detection by their potential prey. Among ceratioid fishes which possess intensely black body pigmentation is the black sea devil *Melanocetus johnsoni,* an angler whose slimy, jet-black skin conceals its presence, contrasting thus with the small, conical, luminous tip of the so-called esca, or waving whiplike lure extending from the animal's snout, above the cavernous, gaping maw, lined with long, sharp, somewhat recurved teeth for capturing any unwary fish which may hover long enough to inspect the dodging, lighted bait lure.

A nearly explosive development of melanin occurs under certain diseased or naturally moribund conditions. Heritable development of melanotic tumors may arise from the presence of abnormal masses of melanophores in a number of fish species and in some reptiles. And there occurs a rapid and extravagant skin-blackening in the Tasmanian whitebait *Lovettia sealii,* following this anadromous fish's spawning activity and its ensuing approach to death as it returns to freshwater. Sexual ripening in this species is accompanied by conspicuously increasing numbers of black skin melanophores, and both sexes, when spawned out—the males notably—display extensive dark patches or, when dying, complete blackening over the whole body surface.

Of conspicuous interest is the demonstration of prompt action by tyrosinase in the nymphal cuticle of the periodic cicada (sometimes called the "seventeen-year locust"), *Magicicada septendecim,* on its emergence from its seventeen-year residence underground (thirteen years in some species). On the nymph's emergence from its underground abode and into the sunlit environment, the biochemical trigger in its special metamorphic metabolism sets off the oxygen-tyrosinase-tyrosine-to-melanin system. The suddenly activated tyrosinase enzyme accelerates the elaboration of melanin, which rapidly darkens the overall body cuticle. If emerging nymphs are immersed at once in previously boiled water previously cooled in a current of inert gas such as nitrogen, and thus now oxygen-free, the generation of dark melanin is precluded; yet it proceeds at once when the insects are exposed to air. Moreover, the water in which the nymphs were immersed now is found to contain both the oxidizing enzyme and the phenolic tyrosine substrate secreted from the insect bodies; therefore, exposure of this water to air evokes its own blackening as well.

Many classes of insects in addition to some which we have considered, possess melanin-darkened wings, wing-covers (in beetles), and body integument.

Rapid melanization, such as in some of the foregoing, has been observed in animal or plant tissues when cut or ground and exposed to air. Such processes emphasize the likelihood of an intimate biochemical relationship between degradation of tyrosine (and of related phenolic derivatives), with ensuing genesis of melanin, and generally accelerated metabolic overturn of protein material. These developments may be associated with the proliferation of new eggs or sperm, with aberrant multiplication of abnormal cells, such as in cancer—involving black moles, or the voiding of blackened urine by patients with melanotic sarcoma, or with extensive degeneration of cellular material in general.

The melanin-laden inks of cephalopods and of the crestfish *Lophotus* have been mentioned. Serious consideration should be given to the possibility that the presence of the dark pigment is merely fortuitous, and may not necessarily serve to screen the ejector's flight from a wary predator. Otherwise what function may be ascribed to the dark color at nighttime, at considerable depths, or in dark caves and other unlighted sites? Moreover, certain deep-living squid species eject a luminescent cloud rather than a dark, inky fluid. It would appear quite plausible, based upon certain private observations, to entertain the alternative idea that the ejected ink, whether black, brown, or even reddish (as the author once observed from an octopus), or a luminous current from a benthic squid, the discharged fluid material may serve a function somewhat similar to that invoked by drawing a red herring across the path of prey fleeing from a dog pack, the pack thus being thrown off the trail by the pungent, substituted scent.

Ink from an octopus (e.g., *Octopus bimaculatus*) emits a rich, rather seminal, musky odor. If a stick, dipped in octopus ink is introduced into a tank harboring a hungry moray "eel," *Gymnothorax mordax,* a mortal enemy of the octopus, or, if instead, a few drops of the diluted ink are introduced into the water, the olfactory stimulus of accompanying chemicals thus afforded the moray is unmistakable as the voracious fish darts about in the tank in search of its prey. If, accordingly, an octopus were to be threatened by such a moray—or by a shark or other natural predator—a promise of equal or greater success of escape would seem to hinge on the intended prey's discharge of ink keeping the attacker feverishly occupied pursuing an olfactory search of the area from which the prey had fled, rather than acting as a mere transient curtain intended to conceal flight. Ejected cephalopod ink is, in any case, apt to assume the form of stringy chains, "blobs," or shapeless coagula in water, rather than a quickly homogeneously dispersed, concealing cloud.

I have conducted additional experiments with octopus ink as an attractant for the moray. The trials focused added evidence upon the role of ink in stimulating the chemical senses. In one test, a mussel, *Mytilus californianus,* dissected from its shell, was offered to a moray, which inspected and tentatively sampled, then dropped it. The same bait, recovered, dipped in octopus ink, and reoffered, evoked the eel's avid seizure and swallowing of it. In another experiment, a small, brownish sea star, *Pisaster ochraceous,* whose externally tough, rigid, and heavily armored body render it altogether without gustatory appeal, was offered the fish. The hungry moray merely ignored the offer. Nevertheless, dipping one of the star's arms in octopus ink and reoffering it to the moray induced immediate and rapid seizure of the dipped arm, with vain attempts to swallow it.

It is difficult to appraise the ink's melanin pigment itself as being anything much more than an adventitious component without odor or taste, and whose color per se must have little to do with the economy or safety of the octopus which secretes the fluid. The accompanying volatile, chemical attractants may, however, serve the animal very usefully as a false, delaying cue during its escape from enemies.

The alluring subject of melanism and the possible biochemical significance attached to it should not be dismissed without mention of another important instance of this pigmentary substance's occurrence and function, lest it remain tacitly labeled as a mere waste-product from the breakdown of tyrosine and allied phenolic compounds, and serving only by chance a role in animals' adaptive concealing coloration or as a screen against injurious sunrays.

Reference should be made to a specialized role played by melanin pigment as a dynamic aid to certain animals' vision. For example, melanin constitutes the dark choroid pigment present in and recoverable from the eye of certain selachian or cartilaginous fishes, especially sharks and some rays. These employ the pigment as a reversible, multicomponent curtain, shading or exposing the light-receptor cells within the retina, in bright or dim light respectively, depending directly upon relative intensity.

Lying directly beneath the white, guanine-laden choroid tapetum lucidum in the eyes of many selachians is a stratum of darkly pigmented choroid cells, which in bright incident light extend multiple strands that aggregate or overlap one another, thus constituting a dark, compound canopy or shield overlying the reflective tapetal elements. In darkness or in subdued light, this process is reversed as the compound curtain is withdrawn, and visual acuity presumably is thereby increased.

Tapetal occlusion of this kind can be induced unilaterally, for example, by exposing one eye of the horned shark *Heterodontus francisci* to bright light while masking the other. The masked eye, now exposed for quick inspection, manifests a bright, unshielded tapetum (nocturnal eyeshine), whereas the previously exposed eye displays conspicuous shielding of its tapetum.

In this typical instance, we encounter the utilization of a waste product, melanin, serving not merely as a protective shield against damaging rays of the sun, as in the integument, or for camouflage purposes in lighted regions, but incorporated as a mobile, readily adjustable system in the visual equipment. As such it operates against dazzle by occluding the retinal receptors, and in promotion of improved vision in dim light by retraction to maximally expose the receptors, whether for seeing predators or prey.

Conceivably a shark, adapting its eyes for enhanced visual acuity in only moderately lighted waters by partially occluding its tapetum, profits at the same time by thus diminishing its otherwise conspicuous eyeshine. At deeper, darker levels, the increased tapetal exposure, augmenting the predator's visual perceptiveness, should more than compensate for any enhancement of potential eyeshine and the fortuitous warning signal the latter might afford.

Melanins are directly functional also in numerous marine invertebrate animals which, possessing no eyes, are equipped instead with photosensitivity in certain integumentary spots or even over whole, diffuse areas of the skin.

A critical and brilliant series of investigations into examples of this, focusing primarily upon the echinoids, carried out by N. Millott and his associates, began about 1950 and extended for many years.

Millott and his colleagues pointed out that echinoids, such as the poisonous-spined form *Diadema antillarum* of West Indian waters, react readily to light or darkness by changing the dispersion of melanin in the pigment cells of the integument. The dark pigment within the melanophores is retracted during nocturnal hours, or when the animals are quartered in a darkened aquarium, when they become very pale. During natural illumination at daytime, or when kept in brightly lighted aquariums, the animals cause their melanophores to spread the dark pigmentary contents, giving the whole body a black color.

These chromatic changes are accompanied by physiological responses involving the animals' spines, as well as the tube feet, which bear terminal sucking discs or paired, clamping jaws for seizing prey. Thus a sudden shading over a part of the urchin's integument will evoke a quick focusing of points of a number of spines in the immediate vicinity, toward the shadow's source. Simultaneously the tube feet become elongated, waving about in the same direction, and the pedicillariae, bearing terminal jaws, may exhibit exploratory motions and clamping action.*

Passing reference should be made here to another class of heteropolycyclic, quinonelike pigments, the so-called ommochromes, which involve oxygen and nitrogen atoms in one or more of their condensed rings. They are thus reminiscent of the melanins, with which pigments they were indeed at one time confused.

The name of this group is from a Greek word for eye, *omma*. These yellow, ruddy, brown, sometimes even black compounds are breakdown products of the amino acid tryptophan, and can be far more colorful than the somewhat related melanins, which arise from the oxidative degradation of tyrosine.

The ommochromes include the ommatins and ommins. The ommatins, fairly complex in chemical structure, still are relatively simple compared with the ommins. An example from the ommatin group is xanthommatin (see App., 53), whose acidic properties are inherent in the pair of carboxylic radicals, as well as in the phenolic group attached to one ring. This is a yellow pigment met with in the molting fluid of the butterfly *Aglais* (*Vanessa*) *urticae.*

Geneticists have utilized, in researches on the fruit fly *Drosophila melanogaster,* the various vermilion, cinnabar, brown, and other eye colors as markers of genotypes. Other insects may exhibit similar eyecolors from the presence of pigments of this same class.

Certain crustaceans' eyes, eggs of a large marine, echiuroid worm *Urechis caupo,* and the rapidly changeable pigment cells in the skin of cephalopods (but not in the case of fishes, reptiles, or amphibians, which have melanophores) also owe their colors to the presence of these compounds.

The ommins are larger molecules, wherein the color-carrying

*The subject has been eloquently discussed by Millott in numerous publications, including three reviews: "Studies on Tropical Echinoderms and Primitive Light Perception," the title of an inaugural lecture at Bedford College, University of London, November 1955; "Animal Photosensitivity, with Special Reference to Eyeless Forms," *Endeavor,* XVI, No. 61 (1957), pp. 19-28; and "The Enigmatic Echinoids," from a symposium, "Light as an Ecological Factor," British Ecological Society Symposium No. 6, Blackwell, Oxford, 1966.

ommatin part is condensed, apparently with longer molecular chains such as polypeptides, or longer amino acid series. The occurrence of ommatins in eyes or skin is not known to be correlated with any role that such pigments might suspectedly play in photoreception or light sensitivity. No physiological function has yet been recognized for these rather limited pigments.

7
Tetrapyrroles: Porphins and Bilins

The needle's eye, it does supply
The thread that runs so true,
The porphyrin thread, blue, green or red,
The living universe through.

(Adapted from an old game-rhyme)

PORPHINS
(App., 54-58; pls. 4, 5, 38-44)

An earlier rhetorical allusion to the green universe of plants, containing and supporting the red kingdom of animals, is not too wide of the mark. For there is indeed a common denominator. It has reference to the fact that the ubiquitous and greatly predominant green colors of the plant world and the widely incident red pigmentation of blood, and hence of animals' skin areas, combs, wattles, tongue, lips, and other mucous areas all manifest the presence of specially structured compounds, the porphyrins, belonging to the tetrapyrrole class of biochromes.

Whereas the porphyrin compounds themsleves possess a cyclic skeleton aggregating sixteen atoms (i.e., twelve carbon and four nitrogen), their relatives, the bilichromes, metabolically allied to them, are of linear conformation, possessing the four nitrogen atoms and the same number of carbons but one, having lost one linking methylene group with rupture of the sixteen-membered ring. These large organic molecules thus are of similar empirical composition and molecular weight; cf. the two red pigments protoporphyrin, $C_{34}H_{34}O_4N_4$, mol. wt. = 562.64, versus bilirubin, $C_{33}H_{36}O_6N_4$, mol. wt. = 584.66, the difference in weight reflecting the loss of one carbon atom, compensated by the gain of two oxygens and two hydrogens (see structural details in App., 56, 62).

While the tetrapyrroles do not occur at high concentrations, their presence is vitally significant to living processes. We have only to exemplify, in the first instance, such common members as chlorophylls, the green porphyrin derivatives which carry out their indispensable role of implementing the photosynthetic generation of carbohydrates from water and atmospheric carbon dioxide. The red porphyrin heme, conjugated with a histone protein, globin, while also chelated to ferrous iron, affords the hemoglobin molecule (mol. wt. ca. 68,000), which serves in the reversible acquisition and transportation of atmospheric oxygen in animals; its somewhat smaller relative, myoglobin (mol. wt. ca. 17,500, or one-quarter that of hemoglobin) likewise serves in the storage of oxygen in red, muscular tissues. Myoglobin involves but one porphyrin unit and one iron atom per molecule, in contrast to hemoglobin's four of each.

There also is a striking example of a vegetable hemoglobin in the root nodules of leguminous plants which harbor symbiotic bacteria of the *Rhizobium* genus. Given accordingly the rather cacophonous cognate name of leghemoglobin, this red biochrome does not serve as an oxygen carrier (hardly imaginably necessary in a green plant in any event), but is biochemically effective in catalyzing the reductive fixation of atmospheric nitrogen, thus giving rise, through an initial hydrazine and/or ammonia synthesis, to various organic nitrogen compounds, including proteins. This process proceeds only in the living tissues, and requires the presence of both the nodular cells and the bacterial symbionts. Hemoglobin may serve yet another extraordinary catalytic function in accelerating the breakdown of hydroxylamine into elementary nitrogen, ammonia, and water in accordance with the equation

$$3H_2NOH \longrightarrow N_2 + NH_3 + 3H_2O$$

The tetrapyrrole skeleton of the chlorophyll type in green plants bears a centrally placed, chelated atom of magnesium instead of iron, as in the heme derivatives. Chlorophyll also bears an additional isocyclic group, condensed upon two neighboring carbon atoms of one of the pyrrole rings; and a long-chained, unsaturated alcohol, phytol ($C_{20}H_{39}OH$), is esterified with a propionic acid side chain attached to a neighboring pyrrole ring (App., 54).

Virtually all organisms, plant and animal, are capable of synthesizing the pyrrole ring, and thus of storing the derived amino acids proline and oxyproline. As we have seen, however, they also are able to effect the binding of such pyrrolic rings, achieving chains or cycles of four such units, each linked to its neighbor by a methenyl (—CH=) group.

Hemoproteins (App., 55; pls. 4, 5, 38)

Hemoglobin, myoglobin, erythrocruorin (from certain marine annelid worms), catalase, and certain other peroxidases carry the same protoporphyrin, with its respective side chains. These differ, of course, with respect to the protein to which the iron-porphyrin moiety is conjugated.

Again, certain metal-complex combinations prevail, for example, magnesium among the chlorophylls, iron in hemoglobin and in the hematin enzymes. Complexes of porphyrins with other metals such as copper and zinc are of natural occurrence, for example, copper uroporphyrin or turacin, the red, alkali-soluble compound in the feathers of the African fruit-eating turaco. This is a pigment without known biochemical function, unless it be to rid the blood of both the metal and the excess porphyrin. Zinc also is known to chelate chemically with some waste prophyrins.

Note has been taken of the fact that iron, bonded as a porphyrin complex, may possess differences in valence. Thus only ferrous (Fe^{++}) iron is functional in the reversible association with molecular oxygen and its transport to the tissues, and in its function as a true enzyme (see below). Peroxidases, including catalase, operative in the release of oxygen from hydrogen per-oxide, bear ferric iron (Fe^{+++}), while the cytochromes and cyto-chrome oxidases exercise their biochemical functions by virtue of the reversible valence of the $Fe^{++} \rightleftharpoons Fe^{+++}$ atoms complexed to the porphyrins.

The nature of the particular protein involved exercises pro-found influence on the whole molecule's function, whether as an oxygen carrier, or as an oxidative or peroxidative agent, or serving to govern the rate and/or extent of oxidation, for exam-ple, between fetuses and mothers, or in gestation among vivipa-rous animal species.

It will be well to cite in this connections an important review, published in 1975 in the *Annals of the New York Academy of Sciences,* occupying all of volume 244, and devoted to "The Biological Role of Porphyrins and Related Structures." Such a modern and comprehensive survey transcends by far, in volume and detail, what may be accorded only passing, or in certain areas even some special, attention in such a treatment as is offered or intended in the present book.

It may be helpful, and perhaps stimulating toward further search by interested readers, to offer a brief outline of the sub-ject matter treated in the cited survey.

Thus there is an early chapter discussing the role of leghemo-globin in the nitrogen-fixing legume root nodules. Another deals with chemical oxidation-reduction reactions of hemopro-teins. Yet another takes up the subject of plant chlorophylls in vivo and their associated proteins. Later coverage is given to porphyrin synthesis from particular approaches. Two chapters deal with porphyria diseases: one on the clinical biochemistry of the human hepatocutaneous kind; the other with comparative aspects of porphyria in man and other animals. An allied chap-ter treats the subject of porphyrins and related compounds as photodynamic sensitizers. There is one chapter which discusses the enzymatic genesis of bilirubin from hemoglobin, through action of a particular heme oxygenase system (which ruptures the porphyrin ring) followed by a reducing enzyme's participa-tion in converting the product to bilirubin. Finally, there are a couple of particularly appealing chapters dealing with compara-tive zoochemical features. One of these concerns red-, white-, and blue-shelled eggs of birds, as models of porphyrin and heme metabolism, a subject pursued earlier by G. Y. Kennedy and H. G. Vevers with eggshells of the Araucana fowl; and finally there appears the most recent coverage of porphyrins in invertebrates, by G. Y. Kennedy of Sheffield, England.

The comprehensive publication is recommended to any specially interested readers who may desire to pursue in depth the subject of porphyrins in general.

We shall accord the porphyrin hemoproteins a passing survey, followed by a similar consideration of miscellaneous unconjugated porphyrins.

Not all cyclic tetrapyrroles are of the same particular configuration or function mentioned above. There are related biocatalysts, such as the cytochromes, as well as other peroxidases, both types fulfilling vital roles in cellular oxidative processes. These are found in protoplasm generally, with some likely exceptions confined to certain anaerobic bacteria. They involve combined iron, but partly in its oxidized or ferric, and partly in the ferrous, state; their porphyrin portions are conjugated with characteristic proteins.

The commonest member, cytochrome *c*, has an iron-bound heme differing somewhat from that of hemoglobin and is easily reduced by mild biochemical reagents. Containing but one hematin unit and one iron atom per molecule, cytochrome *c* carries about 0.43 percent Fe, and shows a molecular weight of about 13,000. The reduced form, ferro*chrome c*, shows more numerous and sharply defined spectral absorption bands in the green, blue, and violet ranges than does its oxidized counterpart, ferri*chrome c*.

Cytochrome *b*, another conjugated hemoprotein, appears to involve a heme (App., 55) identical with that of hemoglobin. In its reduced state, it is slowly reoxidizable by atmospheric oxygen to give ferrichrome *b* without enzymatic mediation. Neither of the two resolvable fractions of cytochrome *a* appears to possess the same heme as that of hemoglobin. All of the cytochromes are red, and are each characterized by definite sets of absorption bands in the visible spectrum. Values for such data are readily available in standard, published tables.

Catalase, an enzyme of nearly universal incidence in living

materials, is a protein conjugated with iron-protohemin as its active group, as in hemoglobin itself, but catalase involves ferric or trivalent iron. This biocatalyst implements the release of free oxygen from hydrogen peroxide. Like hemoglobin, catalase involves four iron-hemin groups, but, being conjugated with a heavier protein, has a much higher molecular weight, ca. 240,000. Other iron-containing hemoproteins, such as the peroxidases, are kindred in basic structure and biochemical function.

A singular additional metal-containing tetrapyrrole compound calls for reference here. This is a vitamin B_{12}, chemically known as cyanocobalamin ($C_{63}H_{88}O_{14}N_{14}PCo$) a red, crystalline compound* synthesized by a number of microorganisms, essential to their normal metabolism and to that of many, if not all, animals. Its tetrapyrrole molecular skeleton closely resembles that of the porphyrins, save for its lack of but one interlinking methenyl group between a pair of pyrrole units (rings A and D). The salient character of this complex molecule is that it involves a centrally placed atom of (trivalent) cobalt (App., 59). Remarkable also is the presence of a cyanide (—CN) radical in the commonest natural form of the vitamin.

Vitamin B_{12} is known medically as the anti-pernicious-anemia factor, since its presence in sufficient (but actually minute) quantities prevents the incidence of that disease and associated disorders such as gastric mucus membrane atrophy and achlorhydria. It also is an extrinsic factor promoting the development of red blood cells in vertebrate animals. There are indeed several forms of vitamin B_{12}, the so-called cobalamins: the differentiating anion attached to the cobalt atom may be hydroxyl, amino, or other alternatives. However, cyanocobalamin, in which the cyanide (—CN) radical is the extrinsic ion ligated to cobalt, is the principal form applied in medicine.

The compound is needed in the diet of man and all other higher animals so far investigated on this point. Some carry in their alimentary tracts the symbiotic microflora which elaborate the vitamin. The compound's primary synthesis resides in certain bacteria and molds, whence, from the intestinal tracts of

*Solubility in water = ca. 1.2 percent at room temperatures; λ_{max} in visible spectrum = 550 nm.

animals, it accumulates in the liver and to a somewhat lesser extent in red muscle, as well as in erythrocytes, and in slight concentrations even in the plasma. Vitamin B_{12} has not been reported in higher plants, and it is interesting to note that pernicious anemia has been observed among so-called "vegans," or extreme vegetarians, wherein it can be relieved, if treated early enough, through the administration of liver and other meats in large amounts.

Pernicious anemia involves a great diminution, even at times a lack, of hydrochloric acid, essential in gastric digestion. Disturbances in the metabolism of iron, zinc, and copper occur, accompanied by aberrancies in numbers, sizes, shapes, and hemoglobin content of the red blood cells. There also may be some psychic disturbances. Deficiency of cyanocobalamin itself, as well as insufficient folic acid (another member of the vitamin B_{12} complex), evoke abnormalities in bone marrow and hence a reduction in red cell production, as well as imbalance between numbers of red and white cells of the blood. Massive doses of the vitamin are effective in overcoming the disease, the recurrence of which may be precluded by continued minor doses.

There are circumstances under which certain porphyrins, present in uncombined condition, may be very toxic. Sometimes, through some metabolic disorder, the processes in tetrapyrrole synthesis become interrupted, or a heme group may become merely detached or split off in some manner and prematurely released instead of proceeding through the usual major sequence of ring rupture, affording the linear or open-chained configuration of the bilichromes. Then such uncombined porphyrin fragments, set free in the blood and other tissues, may accumulate to give rise to pathological conditions known as the porphyrias, a group of disorders, whether heritable or acquired, involving faulty metabolism of the cyclic tetrapyrroles in humans and some other vertebrates.

The two chief biochemical and clinical categories of such diseases are (1) erythropoietic porphyrias, subgrouped into uro-, copro-, and proto-porphyrias, where relatively large amounts of the respective porphyrin compounds are encountered in the normoblastic cells of the bone marrow, and (2) hepatoporphyrias, including acute, intermittent porphyria, so-called variegate porphyria, and porphyria *cutanea tarda*. In these disorders, excessive porphyrins and porphyrin genesis occur in the liver.

The erythropoietic condition involving uroporphyrin is uncommon. It seems to be recessively heritable and involves excessive production and release of type I isomer of porphyrin. Uroporphyrin III (App., 57) is the normal, main product of porphyrinogenesis and is subsequently involved in hemoglobin synthesis. Enzymatic defects may, however, entail greatly magnified elaboration of uroporphyrin I and coproporphyrin I (App., 57-58). Release of such compounds into the circulation leads to porphyrinuria, wherein the pink or red colors of uro- and copro-porphyrin are recognizable in the urine. Alternatively, deposition of such compounds in the skin evokes pronounced sensitivity to sunlight. Rather more rare is the incidence of erythropoietic copro- and proto-porphyrias, wherein such compounds show increased incidence in the red blood cells.

Erythropoietic porphyria is incident early in life, and not many victims reach middle age. Skin lesions and dermatitis are common symptoms, often accompanied by scarring and infection. Other common signs are excessive hairiness, melanotic skin-darkening, and increased mechanical sensitivity of the skin. Hemolytic anemia and spleen enlargement may be incident, as well as red pigmentation of bones and teeth.

In hepatic porphyria, the acute intermittent type probably is heritable as a dominant factor, related to overproduction of porphyrins and their accumulation in the liver. This leads to most distressing, recurring symptoms of pain, nausea, and distention, with diarrhea or constipation. Convulsions may occur, with muscle pain and sometimes sensory loss, often with severe psychiatric manifestations. The urine, usually normally colored, may redden or blacken on exposure to sunlight. The porphyrins responsible may be recognized by their ability to fluoresce under ultraviolet light and by the positions of their spectral absorption bands. An extraordinary fact is that in hepatic porphyria much of the excreted, urinary porphyrin appears as complexes of zinc.

Hemoglobin is sometimes designated by certain alternative

chemical terms, such as ferrohemoglobin or ferrohemin globin, wherein the complexed iron is all in the bivalent or ferrous Fe^{++} state. Oxyhemoglobin may be similarly referred to, save that its name indicates its (reversible) association with oxygen.

In hem*i*globin, variously referable to as ferrihemoglobin, ferrihematin globin, or more commonly methemoglobin, the iron has become oxidized to its ferric or trivalent Fe^{+++} state. This may be effected in the laboratory with common oxidizing agents such as peroxide, ferric tartrate, ferricyanide, bivalent copper ion, nitrates, chlorates, by quinones and other organic reagents, or even by some reducing substances such as cysteine or ascorbic acid in the presence of oxygen.

Methemoglobin will not associate with oxygen or carbon monoxide, as does hemoglobin itself; hence, although not toxic, it cannot support life if present in the blood of a vertebrate. The compound does, however, occur (but not invariably) at minor levels in the ordinary blood of vertebrates studied, for example, about 1.7 percent in man, with similar proportions in blood of the dog, rabbit, and cat, while horse blood may carry somewhat more. Its function, if indeed it has any, has not been recognized; its presence in normal blood likely is metabolically adventitious, resulting from aberrant oxidation processes.

Pulmonary intake of gaseous carbon monoxide (which is odorless) permits this compound to associate with hemoglobin more firmly than does oxygen, hence to displace the oxygen in part. The resulting carboxyhemoglobin is useless in respiration. If present in sufficient amounts, and not discharged soon enough, there may be fatality from asphyxiation. The lips in such cases are characterized by a bright, cherry-red color. Even minor poisoning from limited breathing of CO can lead to very painful, throbbing headache, until protracted intake of fresh air gradually displaces the foreign molecules from their invasion of the blood hemoglobin.*

The various iron porphyrin hemoproteins all are of fundamentally red color, but can be distinguished by spectroscopic examination of the numbers and positions of absorption bands,

---

*This I can recall clearly, it having occurred accidentally to myself one night, during very early morning hours in my third undergraduate year, when I was scheduled that day to sit for two examinations. Not recommended!

principally in the visible spectrum. Some examples are outlined below. Known principal bands are italicized.

Hemoglobin (nonoxygenated): dark (bluish) red: *560* (broad); 430 nm
Oxyhemoglobin: bright red: *577;* 541; 414 nm
Carboxyhemoglobin: cherry-red: *571;* 539; 418 cm
Methemoglobin or ferrihemoglobin: In alkaline media (pH > 9): *600:* 577; 540 nm; in acidic media (pH < 7): *630;* 570; 406 nm
Myoglobin from red muscle: *555;* 475 nm
Oxymyoglobin: *582;* 542; 418; 376 nm
Carboxymyoglobin: *579;* 540; 424; 406 nm
Metmyoglobin: Alkaline: pH > 7: *590;* 540 nm. Acidic: pH < 7: *630;* 500 nm
Catalase: *623;* 536; 400; 280 nm
Chlorocruorin, from polychaete worms, e.g., *Spirographis: 574* nm (broad)
Oxychlorocruorin: *604;* 560 nm
Ferro*cytochrome *c*: *550;* 522; 415; 345; 315 nm
Ferri*cytochrome *c*: *565;* 530; 407; 346 nm

And, for the *cobaltous* tetrapyrrole-ring compound cyanocobalamin, the vitamin B_{12} molecule:

Monocyan compound in water: 550; 361 nm
Dicyan compound in water: 580; 540; 368 nm

The hemoglobins proper are generally recognized as being of wide occurrence in vertebrates (nearly all). It is not present in the primitive chordate *Amphioxus*. Moreover, the parenthetical qualifier "nearly," regarding hemoglobins in vertebrate bloods, has reference to a few notable exceptions among the teleosts or bony fishes. Relatively inconspicuous among examples is the absence of this red blood pigment in the leptocephalous larva of the eel, which does, however, generate hemoglobin with development into the elver stage. Outstanding instances of vertebrate hemoglobin lack are to be found in the so-called icefishes, belonging to the family Chaenichthyidae, of the order Perciformes, most of whose seventeen known species live in the Antarctic, feeding on crustaceans and small fishes. From the South Georgia whaling waters at least three species of icefish, with colorless gills and blood, have been collected, namely *Champsocephalus gunnari, Pseudochaenichthys georgianus,* and *Chaenocephalus aceratus.* Reportedly, a couple of other species, the icefish *Champsocephalus esox* and the so-called "South Georgia Cod," *Notothenia rossi marmorata,* also have colorless blood.

The Danish zoologist Johan Ruud gave special study to freshly collected specimens of the icefish, or crocodile fish, so called for its wide gape [Gk. *chaino,* "gape, or yawn"], *Chaenocephalus aceratus* (pls. 39-40). These are benthic sluggish animals of low metabolic rate, inhabiting the floor of marine waters at temperatures between ca. 2° and -1.7°C. Attaining lengths of some 60 cm and weighing a kilogram or more, these sizable animals possess naked, scaleless bodies, unossified ribs, and completely colorless blood (or perhaps of a very pale yellow, viewed through broad layers), without any traces of hemoglobin (pl. 41). The blood was found to dissolve only from 0.45 to 1.08 ml, with an average value of 0.67 ml, of oxygen, per 100 ml, which amounts to but a twenty-eighth of the capacity of human blood's oxygen-combining level. Manifestly these fishes' low metabolic requirements are met by their ability to absorb dissolved O_2 by mere diffusion through the body wall, gills, and other tissues. Thus, life must proceed close to the margin of asphyxiation. Lacking adequate blood reserves of available oxygen, this fish at once gasps in distress when taken from the water (pl. 40).

Scrutinizing the colored photographs of such a specimen suggests some persistent questions. For example: (1) Notwithstanding the relative dearth of available oxygen dissolved in the body fluids, there still would appear to be enough to permit, whether necessary or not, the oxidative degradation of tyrosine to afford the generation of darkish melanized areas of the integument about the head and forebody. (2) A steady diet of crustaceans, e.g., red krill, and fishes should provide a certain modicum of included carotenoids, common enough even among deep-sea animals; these, when ingested, would be subject alternatively to storage in tissues, complete rejection in the gut, or degradative oxidation, with discharge of color. The whiteness of gills, extensive areas of skin, also of the blood itself certify to the absence of carotenoids, as well as testifying as to the lack of hemoglobin. Thus, do these consumers completely reject carotenoids in their food, or do they utilize some of their limited oxygen supplies for the oxidative degradation (as well as vitamin A production) in metabolizing the assimilated pigments?

Hemoglobins are of wide incidence among the invertebrates, being dominant in annelid worms, occurring in most polychaetes, numerous oligochaetes (e.g., the large pink-and-purplish-colored earthworm *Lumbricus terrestris,* whose red pulsating dorsal vessel can be seen through the body wall), echiuroids, and leeches. They show scattered incidence in other phyla, including, inter alia, certain flatworms, roundworms (threadworms), brachiopods, some holothurian echinoderms or sea cucumbers, and a few crustaceans, insects, and univalved or bivalved molluscs, even certain protozoans.

Not surprisingly, hemoglobins show considerable chemical differences among animal species due to the varying size and character of the protein portion involved. The iron-porphyrin conjugant is identical in the bloods of vertebrates and many invertebrates, although, among the latter, certain tube-dwelling worms in the sabellid, serpulid, and chlorhaemid families carry a green iron-porphyrin, chlorocruorin, which involves a different heme. Nonporphyrin respiratory metalloproteins in certain invertebrates will be reviewed in a later chapter.

A comparative survey of the hemoglobins from various species reveals more similarities than significant differences (save for the wide variations in makeup of the proteins involved) correlative with evolutionary status, but perhaps more significant as to environmental and adaptational requirements. The following comparative features should serve as sufficient illustration: (1) The molecular weight of different invertebrate hemoglobins varies between values from 17,000 to as high as 3,000,000, while blood hemoglobins of mammals, birds, and fishes are characterized by values close to 68,000, and their muscle myoglobins about half this value, or 34,000, thus affording no distinguishing criterion. (2) Isoelectric point (i.e., pH level wherein the proteins show minimum hydration, solubility, viscosity, and total micellar electric charge) varies rather narrowly, between the slightly acidic value of 4.6 and the mildly alkaline level of 7.5. (3) Chemical composition of the protein moiety shows marked variation in the proportion of various constituent amino acids but without any consistent reference to biological classification. (4) Crystallizability and crystalline form appear not to be correlative with phylar position. This is likewise true of (5) the autoxidizability of oxygen affinity of the iron; (6) readiness of denaturation with alkalis and other reagents; and (7) relative affinities of hemoglobin for O_2 versus CO, also revealing no phylar clues.

As an example, the following short list of relative proportions of $HbCO/HbO_2$ at equal partial pressures of the two gases, O_2 and CO, reveals no evaluative correlations.

Animal	$HbCO/HbO_2$ When $pO_2 = pCO$
Branchiomma (polychaete worm containing chlorocruorin)	570
Chironomus	400
Horse	280
Man	230
Arenicola (marine polychaete worm)	150
Tubifex (freshwater oligochaete worm)	40
Planorbis (red freshwater pond snail)	40
Rabbit	40
Root nodules of legumes + Rhizobium bacteria	37
Gastrophilus (bot-fly larval parasite in alimentary tract of horse	0.67
Myoglobins (various species)	28 to 51

Whereas vertebrate hemoglobins are carried in special blood cells, the hemoglobin-bearing invertebrates are divisible into two general classes in this respect. When a definite circulatory apparatus is present, the heme pigments commonly occur freely in the blood proper, separated from the leucocyte-bearing, colorless coelomic fluid. This condition applies generally to worms of the polychaete and oligochaete orders, including some forms carrying the green, so-called chlorocruorin heme pigment, as in *Spirographis* and *Siphonostoma,* where these chromoproteins are free in the coelomic fluid also.

A number of invertebrates that completely lack or possess all but degenerate vascular systems carry their respiratory proteins within corpuscles in the coelomic fluid; examples of these are such polychaetes as *Glycera, Capitella,* and *Polycirrus haematoides,* the echiuroid worm *Urechis,* and the sipunculids *Phascolosoma* and *Sipunculus,* the latter two carrying a different blood pigment, hemerythrin (see Chap. 9).

At least two polychaetes, *Terebella lapidaria* and *Travisia forbesii,* possess hemoglobin free both in their vascular blood and contained within erythrocytes in the coelomic fluid. The blood of the worm *Megaloma pappilicornis* is contained entirely within vessels, and the hemerythrin pigment resides there within corpuscles.

The polychaete worm *Euzonus mucronata,* common in damp, intertidal sand along the Pacific Coast of North America, owes its bright-red and purplish colors to the presence of freely suspended hemoglobin, characterized by properties closely reminiscent of vertebrate hemoglobin, that is, with spectral absorption maxima at 576 and 540 nm in the oxygenated state, and a broad band centering at 565 nm when chemically reduced. The pigment also gives a typical blue color-reaction when treated with the benzidine reagent.

The hemoglobin of this worm is not contained within cells, but is free in the blood fluid, has a molecular weight in the range from 300,000 to 400,000, and is present at a concentration of about 6.2 g per 100 ml of whole blood (cf. such values as 12.6 percent for goats' blood; ca. 14.6 percent for dogs'; and 15.6 percent for human blood). The oxyhemoglobin serves as an adequate store for respiratory oxygen during periods of from 2 to 4 hours, when intertidal anaerobic conditions may prevail within the moist, buried sand bed. Should longer periods of anaerobic conditions happen to occur, or should they be experimentally imposed, as they were in our laboratory, the worms are able to compensate for the condition by adopting an anaerobic type of respiration, releasing succinic and propionic acids in place of the usual CO_2 expired in aerobic conditions.

Other marine burrowing worms such as *Arenicola* and *Urechis* are believed also to utilize their hemoglobin as does *Euzonus,* storing enough oxygen to constitute a reserve for respiratory needs during periods of anaerobic survival in mud.

When colloidally dispersed in invertebrates' circulatory fluid, hemoglobins serve largely in place of the plasma proteins that are effective in regulating the hydrostatic equilibrium or water relations in general, applying to many other species, wherein the hemoglobin is stored within corpuscles.

The oxygen-combining capacity of (free-living) invertebrates' hemoglobin is generally of lower order than that of vertebrates. This capacity increases in the higher vertebrates, and is maximal in certain aquatic mammals such as porpoises, seals, and whales.

Higher concentrations of myoglobins characterize red, active, vertebrate skeletal muscles than are to be found in the paler, less active, synergistic type. Heart muscle contains certain hemoglobins of both molecular sizes, i.e., of molecular weights 68,000 and 34,000. The skeletal muscles of some diving birds are deep red due to myoglobin.

High oxygen-combination capacity has been encountered in a few invertebrate forms added to those cited, such as the insect *Chironomus riparius,* some freshwater crustaceans, *Ceriodaphnia laticaudatus* and *Daphnia magna* (the so-called water flea); also in a freshwater snail *Planorbis corneus,* an echiurid worm *Thalassema neptuni,* a marine anelid *Arenicola marina,* and a freshwater oligochaete *Tubifex.* Such species apparently utilize the oxygen tenacity of their blood hemoglobin for adaptation to aquatic environments undergoing periods of low dissolved oxygen supply.

A number of microcrustaceans beside *Daphnia,* including members of the Notostracha, Anostraca, Cladocera, Conchostraca, Ostracoda, and some parasitic copepods and cirripeds, are reported to carry supplies of hemoglobin dissolved in their blood plasma. This does not apply, however, to larger Crustacea, e.g., Malacostraca, including lobsters, crabs, crayfish, and the like. Their blood yields no detectable hemoglobin, but has instead the nonporphyrinic respiratory pigment hemocyanin, wherein protein is linked to copper ion. Such pigments will be discussed in Chapter 9.

The cosmopolitan brine shrimp *Artemia salina* develops pink blood showing the spectral absorption maxima of hemoglobin if kept for a fortnight or longer in brine at temperatures of from 18 to 20°C, wherein air is dissolved to only some 18 to 20 percent of its saturation level. In contrast, control animals, maintained in continually aerated brine, commonly possess colorless blood, exhibiting no trace of the oxyhemoglobin spectrum. These and some other invertebrates, as also in some vertebrate animals, augment their hemoglobin supplies under conditions involving oxygen deficiency. The water flea *Daphnia,* if inhabiting oxygen-poor waters, increases its supplies of blood hemoglobin, as does *Artemia,* and with several beneficial consequences, for example, (1) increased life-span, (2) enhanced rate and facility of particulate food gathering through increased activity of the thoracic limbs, (3) more energetic and effective swimming, (4) augmented egg production, and (5) accelerated development of embryos, which derive hemoglobin from the parental blood during the egg stage.

We have investigated at La Jolla the pink-colored mantle, gills, foot, and adductor muscle, as well as the ruddy-brown colored brain ganglion of *Tivela stultorum,* the large, edible Pismo clam which thrives, burying itself in the wave-washed sand, along the coast of Southern California. It was found that the water-soluble pigment extractable from its tissues exhibited spectral absorption bands and chemical properties identical with those of typical hemoglobin or myoglobin. Presumably, this burrowing clam must use the oxygen-storing capacity of its limited hemoglobin supplies in a manner similar to that of its neighboring organism, the worm *Euzonus,* storing enough dissolved oxygen to tide itself over until the hour of the next flow. Other self-sequestering molluscs that store myoglobin are the ill-reputed "shipworm" *Teredo* (in its adductor muscle) and the so-called "pileworm," also a wood-boring bivalve, *Bankia seta-*

cea, where the red pigment is concentrated in its posterior adductor muscle and in the heart.

A couple of holothurians deserve some passing notice in view of the spectral properties of their hemoglobins, the mere presence thereof being in fact noteworthy in echinoderms. *Cucumaria miniata* and *Molpadia intermedia* contain, within erythrocytes, hemoglobins showing more redwardly advanced absorption maxima than appear in any vertebrate hemoglobin. Whereas the average positions of the first two a- and β-bands of vertebrate hemoglobins are close to 578 and 540 nm for oxyhemoglobin, and about 559 nm for the reduced form, the respective values for the two sea cucumbers' blood pigments are as follows:

Cucumaria:	Oxidized:	580; 544 nm
	Reduced:	562; 531 nm
Molpadia:	Oxidized:	613; 569 nm
	Reduced:	588 nm

We note here that *Cucumaria*'s a- and β-maxima are a few nm farther toward the red end than in vertebrate blood, but principally that in the reduced condition there still are *two* maxima, the a-member being in fact, at a somewhat higher wavelength than that of the single maximum of vertebrate hemoglobin. And in *Molpadia* hemoglobin the a-band is far up, into the green region, and higher thus than the corresponding maximum of vertebrate blood pigment by some 35 nm, with the β-band about 29 nm higher than that of its vertebrate counterpart. And the reduced blood pigment in this cucumber is in advance of that from vertebrate blood by showing a maximum nearly 30 nm beyond its value.

Investigations have revealed some interesting comparisons between the hemoglobins of vertebrate-host species and those of invertebrate animals which parasitize them. A few examples follow.

A marine fish *Urophysis blennoides,* whose oxyhemoglobin displays an a-maximum centering at 576.5 nm supports a copepod crustacean *Lernocerca branchialis,* which draws blood from its host's gills and itself possesses a hemoglobin with an

a-band but slightly higher than that of the host, at 579 nm.

The nematode *Ascaris*, parasitic in swine, develops a hemoglobin possessing 2500-fold greater oxygen tenacity (in its body wall) and 10,000 times greater (within its parenteric fluid) than that of the vertebrate host's hemoglobin. *Ascaris* thus demonstrates its ability to deoxygenate the host's oxyhemoglobin even at the low oxygen tension that prevails within the mammalian host's gut.

The larva of the botfly *Gastrophilus*, parasitic in the horse's stomach, is another example. Hemoglobin is manifest only at certain stages of this insect's development, becoming finally localized in specialized tracheal cells which exercise a respiratory function. The hemoglobin has a molecular weight of 34,000, or, like the myoglobins, but half of that in the host's blood. Its absorption bands also manifest certain differences in peak positions from those of the host's pigment, and the parasite's hemoglobin exerts a higher oxygen-binding capacity.

The blood-sucking bug *Rhodnius, prolixus* degrades the ingested hemoglobin from the host, mainly into protohematin, but further breakdown products are found in its other tissues. One pigment, parahematin, is passed along, via the bug's ovarian follicles, into the yolk of its developing eggs, giving them a pink color which prevails until transferred into the newly hatched nymphs as bright red masses.

Among other parasites *Pediculus*, the body louse, appears to absorb its primate host's hemoglobin and even to transfer it unaltered into the eggs.

The marine lamprey *Petromyzon marinus*, parasitic during its adult life by sucking the blood of other fishes, possesses a hemoglobin more resembling some of the invertebrate types than that of its host or of other vertebrates. Some of its differences are seen in its molecular weight of 16,700, isoelectric point of pH 5.7 (versus the more alkaline value of 7.4), and some aspects of its amino acid composition.

Some members of the serpulid and sabellid worm families carry hemoglobin, others chlorocruorin, and a few utilize both kinds of biochrome. The genus *Spirorbis* involves species which may be supplied with either one or the other type, whereas *S*.

militaris has colorless blood containing neither. The genus *Potamilla* presents a puzzle in that, while chlorocruorin is the only blood pigment present, *P. reniformis* bears conspicuous concentrations of hemoglobin in its muscles, while *P. stichophthalamos,* inhabiting the same community with it, possesses little. *Serpula* contains both hemoglobin and chlorocruorin in its blood, young animals having greater proportions of the former, and older individuals predominantly the latter type. There are no significant differences in the oxygen-combining capacity between the two kinds of biochrome in these worms.

The a-band of oxychlorocruorin differs somewhat among the various worm species that carry it in their blood. Its value always exceeds that of common oxyhemoglobin, by some 23 nm or more. Some examples are found in *Sabella:* 605.9, *Myxicola:* 605.6, *Spirographis:* 604.8, *Branchiomma:* 602.9, and *Pomatoceros:* 602.5 nm. The chlorocruorins differ biochemically not only in the conjugated proteins involved, but also in the porphyrin type. Some chlorocruorins are of molecular weight as high as 3,000,000. These pigments are the only naturally occurring biochromes whose chemical properties and physiological functions both resemble those of the hemoglobins.

The older name "erythrocruorin," formerly applied to the red blood pigments of many worms and other invertebrates, is falling into disuse in favor of the more appropriate designation of "invertebrate [or species-named] hemoglobin." The latter would seem to be the more logical choice, since, although the proteins involved differ widely, the porphyrin portion of the molecule is the same heme as that in vertebrate hemoglobins.

Many instances of myoglobins are encountered among species of gastropod molluscs, and this is the more striking since these animals possess the nonporphyrin copper-protein complex, hemocyanin, as their oxygen-transporting agent. However, the myoglobins in such species occur for the most part merely in the buccal mass of pharyngeal muscles in the posterior portion of the mouth, extending into the upper part of the digestive tract. These muscles operate the radular "tongue" or horny, scraping rasp used in feeding. The species possessing red, myoglobin-laden buccal muscles likely use the stored pigment as a kind of auxiliary "oxygen bank," particularly in those forms occupying either mud flats, high intertidal areas, spray zones, or rocky coasts. Mud flats are likely to impose anaerobic conditions on animals which bury themselves beneath the surface during low-tide hours, whereas zones exposed for long periods to the air or to mere spray necessitate the inhabitants' protracted closure against the threat of desiccation. This condition limits the animals' intake of oxygen, save during favorable moist periods.

Wheeler North, while a doctoral student in my laboratories many years ago tabulated a useful list of seventeen representative species of such gastropods, which have, during evolutionary development, elected themselves to the classification of oxygen reservists. He showed correlations between the redness of pharyngeal muscles, and thus the richness of stored myoglobin, and the animals' habitats, as well as the weight of the buccal mass in proportion to total body weight.

Let us consider inhabitants of the spray zone, such as the gray periwinkle, *Littorina planaxis,* and of the high intertidal and spray niches, including *L. scutulata,* the smaller species living just below it, the limpets *Acmaea digitalis, A. scabra, A. cassa,* and *Lottia gigantea,* the owl shell. Each of the latter group requires periods of shell closure against exposure, but also possess well-reddened buccal masses comprising from about 1 percent to nearly 2 percent of the total body weight, thus representing high endowments of myoglobin. On the other hand, half a dozen species characteristic of middle to high intertidal zones (including *Tegula funebralis,* the black turban) may be listed that possess ratios of from 2.3 to 3.4 percent for weight of buccal mass in proportion to whole weight, but have little or no evident stored myoglobin, nor pressing need of it. Two accompanying species carry relatively small, lightweighted buccal masses storing noticeable reserves of red myoglobin. Finally, there are some middle-intertidal, low-intertidal, or permanently immersed species which are either possessed of much pigmented pharyngeal muscle, e.g., *Haminoea virescens,* a bubble shell of the mid-intertidal, or which have but small such muscular masses, though of very bright red color, as in the sea hare *Aplysia californica,* a sizable slug exposed at lowest tides. The green

Plates

Schemochromes

1. Abalone shell (*Haliotis fulgens*)
2. *Morpho* butterfly (*Morpho menelaus*)
3. *Selaginella* blue leaves
4. Cassowaries (*Casuarinus* sp.)
5. Mandrill (*Mandrillus sphinx*)

Quinones

6. Purple sea urchin (*Strongylocentrotus purpuratus*)
7. Red sea urchin (*Strongylocentrotus franciscanus*)
8. Sand dollars (*Dendraster excentricus*)
9a. (*Heterodontus francisci*)
9b. Stained teeth of horned shark

Carotenoids

10. Flamingo (*Phoenicopterus ruber*) and spoonbill (*Ajaia ajaja*)
11. Scarlet ibis (*Guara rubra*)
12. Blood serum of flamingo
13. Garibaldi (*Hypsypops rubicunda*)
14. Juvenile Garibaldi
15. Flag rockfish (*Sebastes rubrivinctus*)
16. Sheephead sexes (*Pimelometopon pulchrum*)
17. Swimming crab (*Pleuroncodes planipes*)
18. Spiny crayfish (*Panulirus interruptus*)
19. Kelp crab (*Taliepus nuttallii*)
20. Webbed sea star (*Patiria miniata*)
21. Soft star (*Astrometis sertulifera*)
22. Sunflower star (*Pycnopodia helianthoides*)
23. Sea slug (*Hopkinsia rosacea*)
24. *Flabellinopsis iodinea*
25. *Chromodoris macfarlandi*

26. Red brine pond, with algal flagellate *Dunaliella salina*
27. Plumose anemone (*Metridium senile*)
28. *Pachycerianthis* sp.
29. *Tealia lofotensis*
30. Blue *Velella lata*
31. Purple skeleton of *Allopora californica*
32. Orange yellow *Eugorgia ampla*, a sea fan
33. Lady beetle (*Coccinella* sp.)

Melanins

34. Zebra eel (*Echidna zebra*)
35. Killer whale (*Orcinus orca*)
36. Young lowland gorilla, *Gorilla gorilla* (Jim, born at San Diego Wild Animal Park)
37. Cheetah and cub (*Acinonyx* sp.)

Tetrapyrroles

38. Frigate bird (*Frigata magnificans*)
39. Ice-fish from Antarctica (*Chaenocephalus acertus*)
40. Ice-fish from Antarctica (*Chaenocephalus aceratus*)
41. Colorless blood of Ice-fish
42. Giant conch shell (*Strombus gigas*)
43. Rock snail (*Hexaplex erythrostomus*)
44. Hartlaub's Touraco (*Tauraco hartlaubi*)
45. Blue coral (*Heliopora caerulea*)
46. Red abalone *Haliotis rufescens* (fed on red algae)
47. Blue-shelled eggs of Catbird (*Dumetella carolinensis*)
48. Egg of cassowary (*Casuarius galateus*)

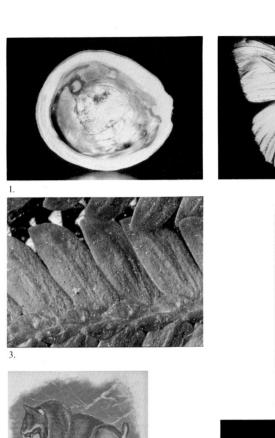

1.

2.

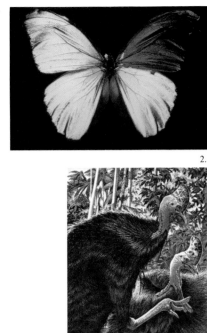

3.

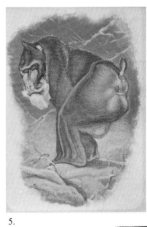

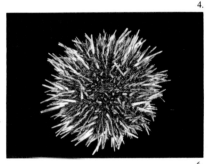

4.

5.

6.

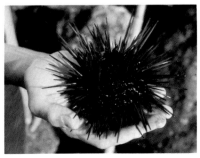

7.

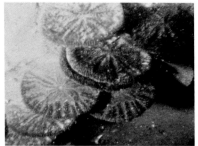

8.

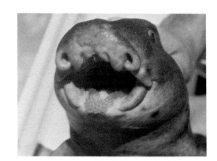

9a.

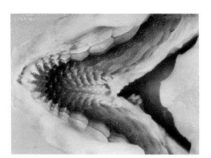

9b.

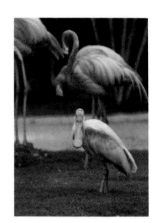

10.

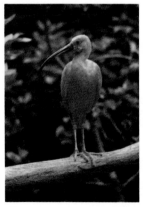

11.

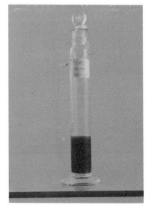

12.

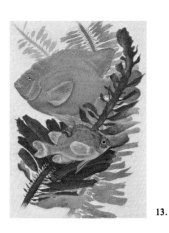

13.

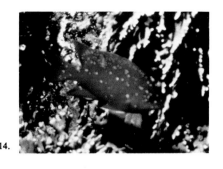

14.

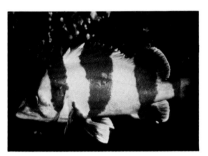

15.

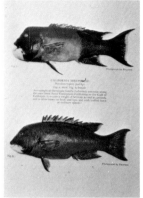

16.

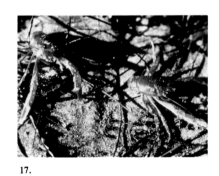

17.

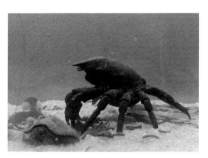

18.

19.

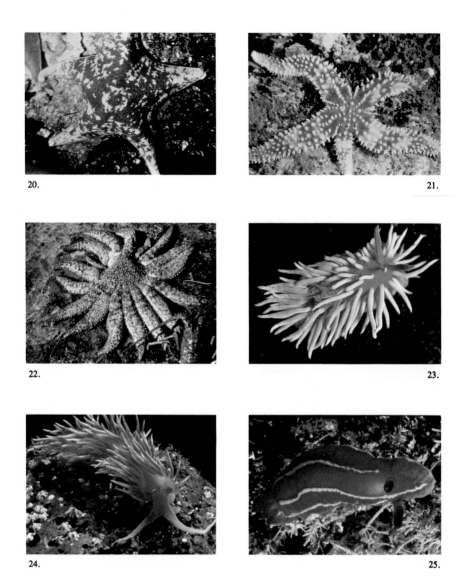

20.

21.

22.

23.

24.

25.

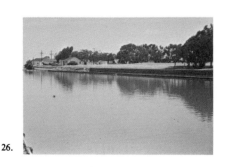

26.

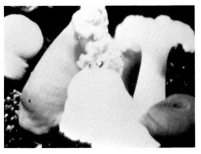

27.

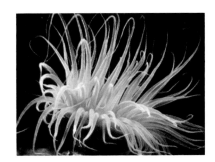

28.

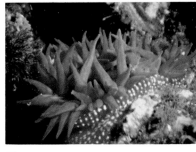

29.

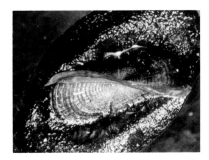

30.

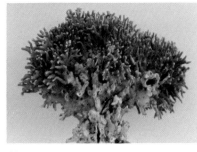

31.

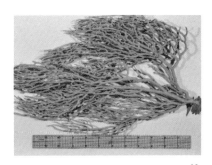

32.

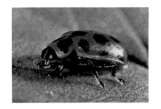

33.

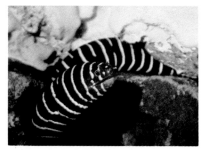

34.

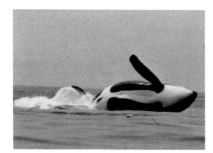

35.

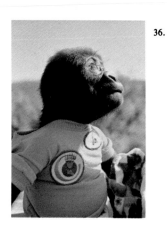

36.

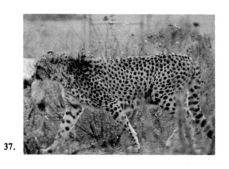

37.

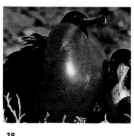

38.

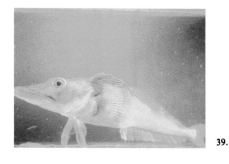

39.

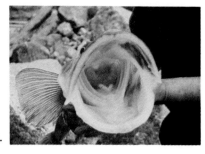

40.

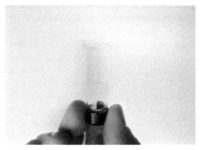

41.

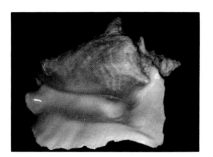

42.

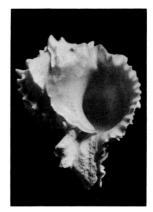

43.

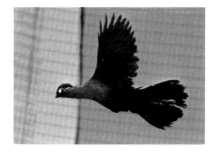

44.

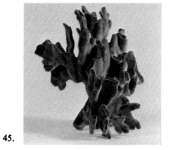

45.

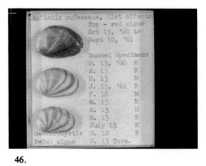

46.

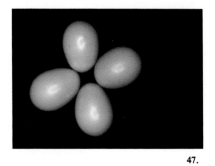

47.

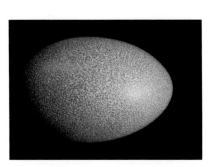

48.

abalone *Haliotis fulgens* possesses only a small pharyngeal muscle mass, but is nearly always immersed in coastal, oxygen-rich waters. The immersed, low-tidal or kelp-inhabiting red turban snail *Norrisia norrisii,* the weight of whose buccal muscles amounts to nearly 2 percent of its total, exhibits pale-colored stores of myoglobin.

The periwinkle, or gray intertidal littorine, *Littorina planaxis,* which needs to store much oxygen for surviving periods of enforced closure against drying of its tissues, has a myoglobin exhibiting typical hemoglobin absorption maxima for the respective oxygenated, reduced, and CO-treated conditions. It differs radically from common hemoglobin, however, in that it dissociates very rapidly from combination with CO when again exposed to air, wherein it quickly combines once more with its normal O_2 complement.

Myoglobins extracted in aqueous media from the pharyngeal muscles of one or more intertidal species of rock-scraping chiton (amphineuran "sea cradles"), have been observed to exhibit absorption maxima closely matching those of common oxyhemoglobin: 578 and 541 nm.

The red pharyngeal muscles and certain digestive tissues of the sea slugs *Aplysia depilans* and *A. limacina* reportedly yield myoglobin of molecular weight 20,000, or heavier by about one-sixth than the usual such macromolecule. Its oxygenated, carbon monoxidic, and ferric derivatives manifest spectral properties in the visible, far-violet, and ultraviolet regions recalling the respective derivatives of mammalian hemoglobin.

Kenneth Read accords a comprehensive survey of mulluscan hemoglobin and myoglobin pigments* He cites researches, including those of Manwell, Prosser and Brown, and Jones, regarding the possible functions of these compounds in the phylum. While the hemoglobin beyond doubt serves to transport oxygen in many molluscan species, it hardly can be regarded as thus serving so limited a function as it does in vertebrates. Such a view receives emphasis and support when one recognizes the seemingly random distribution of these pigments in the molluscan phylum and the absence of heme pigments in

*In Vol. II, of *Physiology of Mollusca,* edited by K. M. Wilbur and C. M. Yonge (1966), Chap. 6.

some species inhabiting environments poor in oxygen supply.

Read provides us with a list of the distribution of molluscan hemoglobin and myoglobin, naming five species of amphineurans, thirty-three gastropods, a scaphopod (the tusk-shell *Dentalium,* which carries radular muscle hemoglobin), and thirty species of bivalves.

Most of the bivalves listed contain their hemoglobin in hemocoelic erythrocytes, or merely dissolved in the hemolymph, whereas the greater proportion of the gastropod species named are characterized by the presence of myoglobin in the radular or pharyngeal muscles. Five planorbid forms, including three species of *Planorbis,* however, carry hemoglobin in the lymph.

An odd hemoprotein of some considerable occurrence among gastropods is the red pigment helicorubin, so named by Sorby, who first identified it a century ago as a pigment recovered from the large terrestrial snail *Helix aspersa.* Manufactured in the so-called "liver," or hepatopancreas, then secreted into the gut by this and numerous other related air-breathing species, the same pigment has been reported to occur also in the digestive gland of the squid *Loligo* and of crayfish.

The absorption spectrum of helicorubin comprises two peaks recalling those of hemoglobin, but shifted instead slightly toward the lower values of λ or wavelength region, by some 6 to 8 units, that is, centering at 571.5 and 533.8 nm. It is, however, a protein protohem*i*chrome, bearing ferric Fe^{+++} iron at slightly acidic pH levels of 5 to 6. In alkaline media (pH 10), the hemo*chrome* form shows stability, and the absorption maxima appear at lower wavelengths: 562.6 and 530.2 nm. The pigment combines only loosely with oxygen or CO but always in acidic media. The animal's respiratory needs are commonly met through its supplies of hemocyanin, although it may risk some oxygen shortage when it seals its operculum in dry environments or at unfavorable temperatures. No physiological function has been established for helicorubin, unless its loose association with oxygen in acidic media may serve for limited storage of the gas against respiratory needs during periods of increased localized acidity through greater CO_2 concentrations generated by the snail during seasonal periods of shell closure.

Miscellaneous Animal Porphyrins*

Wide and varied surveys have been carried out concerning por-
phin derivatives, notably with respect to their chemical and biochemical attributes, whether or not closely related to those of
the heme class.

There are acceptable reasons for the view that tissue porphyrins are not to be regarded only as normal intermediates in the
disintegration of hemoglobin, but possibly indeed in its synthesis. Porphyrins have been encountered in the albumin of the fertilized hen's egg during early developmental stages where the
observed quantities could not have arisen from the small modicum of hemoglobin then present in the embryo. Greater quantities of porphyrin occur in the embryonic blood precursors than
in the erythrocytes themselves, and they increase with accelerated hemopoietic or blood-generating activity in the bone
marrow.

The sixteen-membered tetrapyrrolic rings, interlinked by
their four included methylene chains, differ one from another
merely through the kinds of chemical radicals or side chains carried by attachment to the outer four pairs of carbon atoms of
the respective pyrrolic groups. Indeed, some pairs of compounds are merely so-called isomers, carrying the same kinds
and numbers of such side chains, but with one or more pairs
occupying "exchanged" positions in the overall molecule. Such
isomers have by definition the same empirical formula and
molecular weight and share most of their chemical (but often
not their *bio*chemical) properties, as we shall see.

Among the more common porphyrins are protoporphyrin
(App., 56), one of the earlier-discovered members, occurring in
a few vertebrates and numerous invertebrates, and carrying
four methyl ($-CH_3$), two unsaturated vinyl ($-CH = CH_2$) and
two propionic acid side chains ($-CH_2COOH$). Hematoporphy-

---

*In ensuing discussions under this general heading, it will be impossible to avoid the
application of certain longish chemical names, perhaps not familiar to every reader, for
more important members of the naturally incident porphyrin compounds. Accordingly,
some very brief characterization of some typical examples is called for in passing. Any
readers who might like to see or review the accepted structural formulas of the several
porphyrins considered should refer to the Appendix in the back of this book.

rin, early recovered as the protein-free derivative of vertebrate blood and of wide occurrence throughout the animal kingdom, bears the same number of methyl groups (and in the respective positions), as does protoporphyrin but differs from it in substituting, for the vinyl radicals, a pair of propanolic (or propyl alcoholic) side chains.

Uroporphyrins I and III derive their name from their original isolation from urine, notably in that of patients with porphyria, who void pink-colored urine. The two coproporphyrin isomers I and III had similar historical beginnings. Coproporphyrin I was first detected in feces (hence the name, from the Greek word, *kopros,* "dung"). Uroporphyrin III was first recovered from the urine of a patient with chronic porphyria and later found to be identical with the porphyrin compound, chelated with copper, in red quill feathers of the African fruit-eating touraco, for example, *Tauraco leucotis donaldsoni,* hence called turacin in its copper-complexed state (pl. 44).

The two uroporphyrins possess exactly the same empirical chemical formula ($C_{40}H_{38}O_{16}N_4$), bear the same set of side chains, and are of identical molecular weight: 830.73. They differ from each other solely as to the alternative sites upon which one methyl and one propionic acid group are placed on one or other of a pair of neighboring pyrrolic rings, as shown in the Appendix (57, and see further below).

Similarly, the pair of coproporphyrin isomers (compounds of the same empirical formula $C_{36}H_{38}O_8N_4$) share the same possession and respective numbers of methyl and propionic acid radicals and a common molecular weight of 654.69. Here again, their differentiation is based solely upon the molecular attachment sites of one methyl and one propionic acid group (App., 58).

Of these two general types of excretory porphyrins, the uroporphyrins are the more acidic, bearing eight acid radicals (four acetic and four propionic), versus the presence of but four propionic acid groups as side chains of the coproporphyrins. Uroporphyrins are indeed convertible into corresponding coproporphyrins by chemically removing the four acetic groups, that is, reducing them to methyls.

Readers may review, at their option, the summarized characterization of the more common porphyrins and their side
chains, bearing in mind the legend below (after Lemberg and
Legge, 1949). The Appendix will show the molecular architecture proposed for the respective compounds.

M   = Methyl (-CH$_3$)
E   = Ethyl (-CH$_2$-CH$_3$)
V   = Vinyl (-CH=CH$_2$)
EOH = Ethyl-alcoholic or hydroxyethyl (-CHOH-CH$_3$)
Ac   = Acetic acid (-CH$_2$-COOH)
Pr   = Propionic acid (-CH$_2$-CH$_2$-COOH)
H   = Hydrogen

Porphyrin	*Empirical Formula*	*Side Chains*
Etioporphyrin	$C_{32}H_{38}N_4$	4 M; 4 E
Mesoporphyrin	$C_{34}H_{38}O_4N_4$	4 M; 2 E; 2 Pr
Protoporphyrin	$C_{34}H_{34}O_4N_4$	4 M; 2 V; 2 Pr
Deuteroporphyrin	$C_{30}H_{30}O_4N_4$	4 M; 2 H; 2 Pr
Hematoporphyrin	$C_{34}H_{38}O_6N_4$	4 M; 2 EOH; 2 Pr
Coproporphyrin	$C_{36}H_{38}O_8N_4$	4 M; 4 Pr (App., 58)
Uroporphyrin	$C_{40}H_{38}O_{16}N_4$	4 Ac; 4 Pr (App., 57)

The free porphyrins are amphoteric compounds in that they
have the capacity to serve either (and more often) as acids, com-
bining with alkaline ions to yield salts via their carboxylic acid
radicals, or as bases through their ability to provide acid salts,
involving two of their four nitrogen sites, on treatment with
strong mineral acids such as hydrochloric. Their limited solubility in pure water provides systems of mildly acidic character,
affording pH values ranging between about 3 and 4.5, save for

etioporphyrin, which has no acidic side chains. Most porphyrins are soluble in organic solvents such as ether, save for the uroporphyrins, whose eight acidic terminal groups render them relatively polar compounds, preferentially soluble in aqueous media. The free compounds, and their alkaline and acidic salts, all exhibit characteristic multiple absorption maxima.*

Aberrant or otherwise unusual features of porphyrin formation give rise to such symptoms as (1) the deposition of uroporphyrin in bones and its excretion in the urine, for example, in the case of the fox squirrel *Sciurus niger,* (2) disturbances in the linking of porphyrin with iron, evoking excretion of coproporphyrin, notably in cases of lead poisoning, and (3) biochemical departures from the normal hemoglobin breakdown processes resulting in the release of porphyrins instead of bilins (see discussion of porphyria).

Porphyrins, whether free or combined with metallic ions, are of normal occurrence in very low concentrations in tissues of many animal species, or at higher levels in certain animal products (e.g., feathers, eggshells, molluscan shells).**

There are many instances of differences between the metabolism of uroporphyrins I versus III, or of the corresponding pair of coproporphyrin isomers. Of these, only a few examples will be cited here.

Animals injected with certain porphyrin solutions, or animals and human patients encumbered with chronic porphyria, when exposed to sunlight or ultraviolet light suffer local destruction of the skin, and, under some conditions, death in shock may ensue.

In animal experiments, for example, uroporphyrin I has been observed to be strongly active, coproporphyrin less so, and proto- and hemato-porphyrins only slightly active or harmless.

---

*These are all to be found listed in biochemical handbooks, e.g., *Biochemisches Taschenbuch,* by H. M. Rauen, 1964, as well as in the comprehensive book by Lemberg and Legge, cited earlier.

**A good survey of what has been published concerning the porphyrins in invertebrates is to be found in G. Y. Kennedy's article in the previously cited Annals of the New York Academy of Sciences in 1975. He carries the history of such studies back to 1874, when C. A. MacMunn's investigations on the subject began, and 1877, the year when H. N. Moseley published his first studies on the pigments of certain corals, anemones, and jellyfish.

Moreover, uroporphyrin III was found to be photodynamically inactive, in contrast to uroporphyrin I; coproporphyrin III was assessed as less active than its I isomer.

The amazing fact is that, in such compounds, only minor chemical differences are known. Uroporphyrin I carries its acetic radicals on carbon atoms 1, 3, 5, and 7, and its propionic acid groups on positions 2, 4, 6, 8 (App., 57). Contrastingly, uroporphyrin III, of identical empirical formula and molecular weight, has its four acetic residues on positions 1, 3, 5, and *8,* and its propionic groups at sites 2, 4, 6, and *7* (App. cit). This represents merely a kind of "trade-off," between the otherwise completely identical isomers, of an acetic for a propionic radical on two respective, adjacent carbon atoms in a common pyrrole ring! It will be remembered that the two isomers exhibit the same solubilities in various reference fluids and the *same spectral absorption maxima.* The only recognized differences seem to reside in minor dispositions in the needlelike crystals of the two pure compounds' ectamethyl esters, and a departure between the melting points of the respective esters, that of uroporphyrin I at 290-293° being some 35° higher than the level attributed to uroporphyrin III, at about 255-257°. The comparative biochemist continues to wonder just why, of these two isomers, I is profoundly active physiologically in the presence of sunlight, and III not so at all. Also, why both sexes of the brightly colored touraco secrete into their feathers the red copper complex of uroporphyrin III, supposedly the photodynamically harmless isomer.

We shall undertake next a brief survey of examples of porphyrin-bearing invertebrate animals.

Coelenterates. Actiniochematin, yielding a hematoporphyrin seemingly identical with that derived from hemoglobin itself, was early recognized by MacMunn, about a century ago, in numerous marine actinarians, including color variants of the anemone *Actinia equina,* also of *Tealia felina,* and even the white genotype of *Metridium senile.* The compound has since been compared very closely with cytochrome *b* and with parahematin. Its occurrence is pronounced in muscular tissues of such anemones as *T. felina, Hormathia coronata,* and *Cereus pedunculatus,* and in minor amounts in the muscularly weaker species *Anemonia sulcata, Actinia equina, Adamsia palliata,* and *Cerianthus membranaceous.*

While hardly to be regarded as of any direct respiratory significance in this animal phylum, the porphyrins may conceivably serve in certain metabolic oxidation processes (see cytochromes).

Free protoporphyrin IX has been detected in certain jellyfish and medusae of deeper ocean waters, including *Atolla wyvilli* and *Periphyta periphyta,* but not in either of two shallow-water forms *Pelagia,* the venomous purple jellyfish or *Aurelia,* the active white one.

Two species of sea pen, *Pennatula borealis* and *Balticina finmarchica,* have been found to be pigmented chiefly by protoporphyrin IX, rendering these animals' soft parts highly photosensitive. In *P. aculeata,* however, only very small amounts of porphyrin were detected. These species live on the sea floor, burrowing into it with the stalk, at moderate depths, and hence receive relatively minor amounts of filtered light. It has been suggested that porphyrins, most conspicuous in the tentacles, may serve to guide the animals against migrating into shallower, hence more lighted environments.

Platyhelminthes (flatworms). The well-recognized photosensitivity of planarians such as *Dugesia dorotocephala* may be attributed to the presence of uroporphyrin and coproporphyrin. Affiliated species such as *D. tigrina* and *D. gonocephala,* as well as *Cura foremanii,* all have yielded uroporphyrin of unspecified isomer, while three species of *Phagocata,* as well as *Bdellocephala brunnea,* all yielded an unspecified coproporphyrin. Unidentified porphyrins were recognized half a century ago in the parasitic cestode *Tetrathrydium,* which infests the hedgehog, and in the larval stage, the tapeworm *Taenia solium.* Such prophyrins may likely be derived through the parasites' digestion of hemoglobin ingested from the host.

Annelida (and associates). Under this heading, Kennedy has considered the incidence of various pigments in members of the five chief classes within the annelid phylum, devoting nearly sixty pages to details and some passing mention of some eight-score worms, whether by species or merely families and orders in some cases. Anent these we read of some forty-four named species among which porphyrins occur (excluding instances where the hemoproteins are the only kind specified, since they were considered above). And of those cited,* some porphyrins are of provisional or questionable identity.

Among interesting occurrences of worm porphyrins may be cited the so-called sea mouse *Aphrodite aculeata,* singularly conspicuous for its long, lateral, schemochromically and beautifully iridescent chaetae, or bristles. This large worm bears hemoglobin in its pink pharyngeal muscles and in the crimson nerve ganglia. Accompanying methemoglobin in its alimentary tract are, in the gut contents, protoporphyrin IX, uroporphyrin III, coproporphyrins I and III, and some other related compounds of porphyrin character.

Glycera convoluta and *G. alba* possess a hematin in the gut; and phaeophorbide *a* (the magnesium-free, phytol-free residue from degradation of chlorophyll *a*) as well as coproporphyrin III occur in the gut wall of the aptly named varicolored polychaete *Nereis diversicolor.*

The large mud-burrowing "lugworm" *Arenicola marina,* popular among fishermen as fish bait, was found by Kennedy and Dales to possess pink skin while young, whereas in older specimens this tissue became dark brown or black. Much of both coproporphyrins, but chiefly the III-isomer, was recoverable from the body wall of older, dark-skinned specimens, while less of such material was evident in the skin of the younger, pink individuals. The species yielded uroporphyrin III as well as the coproporphyrin pair of isomers.

Two echiuroid worms, *Bonellia viridis* and *Thalassema lankesteri,* possess a bluish-green porphyrin in the skin and mucus which attracted the esthetic attention of naturalists many decades before it was given some careful study and found to be identical with, or very closely related to a chlorophyll degradation product, mesopyrrochlorin.

---

*In his most recent review Kennedy (1975), cited four polychaetes, three oligochaetes, and an echiurid *Bonellia viridis,* as yielding varying porphyrins; he also instanced Needham's report (1974) of porphyrins in a number of leeches. It seems from what Kennedy had to say that porphyrins have not been reported in any save the one echuroid, nor in typical gephyrian, priapulid, or phoronid worms. Most of his paper indeed deals with carotenoids, melanins, and other biochromes encountered in the annelid worm phylum.

Protoporphyrin has been identified in the pinkish, hemoglobin-bearing earthworm *Lumbricus terrestris,* and an allied form *Eisenia foetida.*

A tube-building polychaete *Chaetopterus variopedatus* bears a dark-green pigment in its intestinal epithelium; long called chaetopterin, it was contained inside small spherules within the tissue. These pigment aggregates involve a number of porphyrins, principally phaeophorbides *a* and *b,* in that order of prominence, derived doubtlessly from the breakdown of the respective chlorophylls *a* and *b.* There is present yet another fraction referred to by Kennedy as an *iso*phaeophorbide *d,* dioxymesophyllochlorin, which is an acidic rhodoporphyrin derivative, and a copper complex of phaeophorbide, along with coproporphyrin III and a trace of another porphyrin bearing *five* acidic side chains.

A red nematode *Eustrongylus gigas,* parasitic in the dog, carries proto- and copro-porphyrins as adventitious breakdown products derived from its host's hemoglobin.

Mollusca. Considering the great numbers within the five classes under this phylum, also their diversity in size and structure, it is perhaps surprising to encounter so relatively few reports on the occurrence within them of free porphyrins, which may be supposed to represent the world's earliest species of colored, biochemically active organic molecules. Of those molluscs that manifest porphyrins, a fair share carry major proportions of these biochromes in their shells, accompanied therein by their close relatives, the linear tetrapyrroles or bilins (see below).

Concerning the gastropods, reports cite porphyrins exhibiting fluorescence, notably under ultraviolet light, in the integument of the terrestrial slugs *Arion rufus, A. ater,* and colored variants of *A. empiricorum.* From the skin of the marine nudibranch slug *Durvaucelia plebia* and from that of two marine tectibranch slugs, the sea hare *Aplysia punctata* and *Akara bullata,* Kennedy and Vevers recovered uroporphyrin I. Kennedy showed that this pigment in the skin of the black garden slug *Arion ater* occurs in quantities directly proportional to the content of dark melanin pigment, which may serve as a screen against injury lest incident sunlight impinge upon the photodynamic porphyrin isomer.

In some early researches on the Pacific Coast cephalopod *Octopus bimaculatus,* S. C. Crane recovered murky green porphyrinlike biochromes from the large so-called "liver" (actually the digestive and secretory hepatopancreas), after the animals had been fed upon hemoglobin-rich diets such as horse or hog liver. The recovery of such a pigment and its chemical and spectral characteristics are discussed in *Animal Biochromes.*

Conchoporphyrin is a name applied to a member of the porphyrin series differing from uroporphyrins, which carry eight acidic radicals, and from coproporphyrins, supplied with but four. Conchoporphyrin, so named from its recovery from molluscan shells, is similar to a coproporphyrin save that it possesses five carboxylic acid side chains; indeed it can be converted into coproporphyrin by the chemical removal of CO_2 from its molecule, thus leaving but the four lateral groups.

Like conchoporphyrin, uroporphyrins are to be found in shells of numerous bivalves and gastropod molluscs (pls. 42-43). Indeed the uroporphyrins are the chief members present, despite the wide genetic variation in color and color pattern. Moreover, the shell porphyrins often are accompanied by conspicuously colored bilins, as we shall see.

Alex Comfort has provided a list of forty-two present-day molluscan forms whose shells involve relatively large amounts of bonded porphyrins, chiefly uroporphyrin I. Of these, twenty, or nearly half, are marked as having this property widespread through several species of a genus.

The chemical stability of porphyrin molecules, once formed, is truly remarkable. Comfort lists, for example, ten fossilized shells from among the Recent British Mollusca demonstrably known to have deposited shell porphyrins. He names also a few much older forms in whose fossil shells porphyrinic fluorescence has been demonstrated, for example, *Gibbula cineraria* from post-Pleistocene times, *Pteria media* from London Clay, and *Fissurella squamosa, Angaria calcar, A. lima,* and *Testus crenularis,* from Upper Eocene measures.

The origin and physiological role of porphyrins in molluscs remain obscure, since these compounds are not, as in the higher forms, associated in molluscs with the formation of hemoglobin via protoporphyrin. They may, however, occupy a place in the elaboration or metabolism of such tetrapyrrolic biocatalysts as the cytochromes or peroxidases. Still why should so many side products be secreted from the mantle and other body tissues and into the shell material?

Some Japanese researches of thirty years ago and longer led to the discovery of varying traces of porphyrins, some of them combined with metals, in colored oyster pearls. Green pearls were found to contain greater proportions of metalloporphyrins (0.033 mg%) compared with metal-free ones (0.015 mg%) than seemed to prevail in pink pearls (0.011 and 0.016 mg%, respectively).

The free porphyrins exhibit arresting red fluorescence, as do their salts, which, in colored pearls, seem to involve lead or zinc. Whatever may be the biochemical origin of molluscan porphyrins, the suggestion has been made that there may be an intimate relationship between calcification and the elaboration, metabolism, and secretion of porphyrins by molluscs. It would seem, however, that since there are many pigment-free pearls and shells secreted by these animals, and moreover, many instances of porphyrin manifestation in shell-less species, such a possible role to be played by mere traces of porphyrin in the elaboration of shell material should be regarded with some reserve.

Echinoderms and Crustaceans. Free porphyrins have been reported by Kennedy and Vevers in only three of some fourteen echinoderm species investigated, viz., the sea stars *Astropecten irregularis, Luidia ciliaris,* and *Asterias rubens.* The integument of the first two yielded chlorocruoroporphyrin and protoporphyrin, while the third species carried in its skin only the latter.

The same investigators encountered no red fluorescence of porphyrins in the tissues or shell of eight marine crustacean species.

Fishes. Certain fish species reportedly contain porphyrins in skin, nerve, and scales. Older workers such as Francis, in 1875, reported what he believed on spectroscopic evidence to be porphyrin in green and blue-green scales of the wrasses *Odax radiatus, O. frenatus,* and *O. richardsonii;* and Wagenaar, in the latter 1930s likened the absorption spectrum of the green nerve cord in the sea pike *Belone belone* to that of a reduced heme. All such surveys deserve to be repeated with a particular view to adding a careful examination for biliverdin.

Birds. When turning to the avian class, it is of special interest to recall a few instances of porphyrin manifestation in the feathers of some species, as also in the eggshells of many.

The quill feather of a touraco, *Tauraco leucotis donaldsoni,* placed in water rendered even barely alkaline, for example, through adding a few drops of ammonia solution, rapidly yields its store of the copper complex of uroporphyrin III as a bright magenta-red solute that affords typical, conspicuous spectral absorption bands at ca. 565 and 528 nm. Rendering the system neutral or even slightly acidic precipitates all of the pigment in red flocks.

Coproporphyrin III has been recovered from feathers of bustard-related birds, such as *Lophotis ruficresta ruficresta, L. r. grindiana,* and *Lissotis melanogaster.* A uroporphyrin compound of some kind has been suspected through the manifestation of fluorescence in the feather shafts of young pigeons, in spines of the hedgehog, and even in the teeth of some mammals.

Of rather special interest is the extensive manifestation or recoverability of tetrapyrrolic pigments from the calcareous material of birds' eggshells. Here again, Kennedy and Vevers have contributed the definitive reports on this subject, deriving mostly from their own researches. They remind us of the fact that the Araucana Fowl (*Gallus domesticus*), found among the domestic poultry in South America (perhaps originally imported there from Asia by the Dutch), deposit eggs varying widely in shell color, for example, from bluish through blue-green, purplish, greenish, gray-green, to green speckled with brown. Kennedy and Vevers were able to obtain 500 g of Araucana eggshells from Whipsnade Park, varied as to color from a dull green-brown to pale blue, many of which, viewed under u.v. light, exhibited red fluorescence.

Extraction of the shells with a methanolic sulphuric acid yielded a bright-blue solution. Dilution and shaking with chloroform effected the transfer of all pigment to that solvent. When free of residual acid, the chloroform solution was evaporated to dryness, the residue redissolved in fresh chloroform, and the pigments were resolved by chromatographic passage through a column of magnesium oxide, whereby four colored fractions were recovered. The presence was established of protoporphyrin, biliverdin, the latter's zinc-chelated complex, and coproporphyrin I. The authors suggested that, since the porphyrin arises from the same cells as the calcium ions, it might play a role in the calcification processes laying down shell material. We are left with the fact, however, that many birds lay white-shelled eggs which carry no porphyrin.

In an extensive survey of avian eggshell pigments, the same team of productive authors examined eggshell pigments from 108 species, for size, color, general appearance, and pigmentary content. Their findings are given in tabulated form occupying five pages. The appearance and colors of the shells are described in such terms as white, off-white, cream, and blue colors, green hues, blue-greens, brown shades including speckles, olive tints, beige, rosy buff, pinkish (brown-speckled), red-brown spots, and other mixtures. The pigments encountered proved to be protoporphyrin (App., 56), biliverdin IX_a (App., 61), and the zinc-chelated complex of the latter compound. All samples were examined for u.v.-evoked fluorescence.

Throughout the overall lot there was considerable scattering of pigmentary properties. Fluorescence was evoked in fifty-two species; of these all showed protoporphyrin also, save that this was not actually recovered in a couple of psittacine species (ring-necked parrakeet and roseate cockatoo), which were among those that lay white-shelled eggs. Perhaps two dozen or thirty species are listed variously as having white, off-white, or cream-shelled eggs.

Of the total, a hundred species laid eggs whose shells contained porphyrin: forty-nine carried this pigment only, another thirty-three had the porphyrin combined with biliverdin, an additional lot of seventeen had shells yielding protoporphyrin and both biliverdin and its zinc-complex, and finally one species yielded only porphyrin and the zinc-chelated biliverdin. Five species had no pigment, while two had biliverdin only; but its zinc chelate never was encountered alone. The authors summarized their findings in a brief table like the following, where P = protoporphyrin, B = biliverdin, and Z = zinc chelate of biliverdin.

Number of Species Examined	P, B, & Z	P only	B only	Z only	P + B	B + Z	P + Z	Nil
108	17	49	2	0	33	1	1	5

Thus the porphyrin component was by far the dominant one, although in the hundred species depositing it in their shells, that is, 92.6 percent of the total number analyzed, only fifty-two manifested fluorescence.

Protoporphyrin (App., 56), earlier called oöporphyrin, occurring as we have seen in the shells of many bird species, is found also in the hen's egg membrane and is demonstrable as well in blood erythrocytes by its fluorescence. Kennedy and vevers reported, furthermore, that the shell of the common gull's egg (*Larus canus*) bears so much protoporphyrin on its outer surface that it may be scratched off readily by a fingernail. Such a condition is reminiscent of occasional observations relating to domestic poultry, such as in the case of the eggshell of a duck and brown-shelled eggs of various breeds of barnyard hens.

An instance of this latter occurrence was reported by Hutt and Sumner, who encountered it in the shell of an egg taken from the oviduct of a four-year-old hen which had been slaughtered for table use. The eggshell bore a substantial rough, granular, dark-brown-colored coat covering the original lighter-brown surface. This protoporphyrin-incorporated layer, containing some protein and calcium salts, was about 1.6 mm thick, and weighed about 12 g. It was concluded that the delay of some weeks of the egg within the uterus and oviduct had entailed no additional deposition of calcium into the shell proper, but had allowed the uterine pigment deposition to continue for the abnormal period. The avian uterus (not considered as being homologous with the mammalian uterus), reportedly contains small, brownish, granular porphyrin within its epithelial cells.

The red fluorescence characteristic of porphyrins has long been a metabolic sign in the avian class, having been reported in the shells of fossilized eggs from the Tertiary period and having thus persisted over some millions of years.

In warm-blooded vertebrates, both birds and mammals, there

is porphyrin in the white matter of the brain, spinal cord, and certain other related nervous tissues. Hematoporphyrin has not been demonstrated there, but coproporphyrin, perhaps both I and III, and probably, smaller proportions of protoporphyrin have been reported. Observations respecting these were first made on humans and other warm-blooded animals by fluorescence spectroscopy in situ, as well as through the examination of extracts. The porphyrins seem not to be present at birth, but to appear in the spinal cord at about three weeks of age in rats, after about eight weeks in ducks, and to develop still later in the brain. Klüver, who reported earlier on this work, mentioned the appearance of a striking and well-defined emission band in the red region at 620 to 630 nm, with a maximum at 625 nm, when white nervous tissues of twenty-five species of mammals and birds were examined under light from a mercury-vapor source, passing first through a suitable Corning glass filter. None of eight species of amphibians and reptiles manifested the fluorescent biochrome.

The warm-bloods studied were mammals including man, green-, cebus-, spider-, and squirrel-monkeys, brown bat, cat, dog, guinea pig, rat, mouse, pig, sheep, goat, hartebeest, Grant's gazelle, ox, and opossum; and birds including the common rhea, duck, chicken, pigeon, and great horned owl.

The adult group of cold-bloods included the fully grown leopard frog, bullfrog, iguana, Gila monster, and the Texas-collared, bull, indigo, and milk snakes. Referring to the warm-bloods, Klüver remarked on the higher concentration of porphyrins in the central nervous system than elsewhere in the body, and upon its increase with the advance of adulthood. He suggested that neurological and psychiatric disorders may reflect a "cerebral porphyria" under some conditions.

It has been observed that estrus, coincident with female and male development and egg-laying, is stimulated by length of day, that is, maximal exposure to incident light. Not only are duration and intensity of exposure notably effective, but fractions of certain wavelengths conjoin, in promoting reproductive activities in normal vertebrates. Photostimulation of sexual activity is strongly triggered by incident red or orange light, less so by yellow, and little if at all by green, blue, or violet. This was demonstrated by Benoit and Ott longer than thirty years ago: exposure to red, orange, or yellow rays evoked accelerated testicular development in immature drakes via initial impingement upon the retina, thence stimulating the hypophysis, and thence further the gonad. Indeed, when led directly through a quartz rod onto the hypophysis of enucleated birds (i.e., the eye proper having been removed), even blue-violet rays, which evoke little if any stimulus under normal conditions, were observed to equal or exceed in their effects the red rays similarly introduced. Short rays of the blue and violet regions are filtered out by the tissues, bones, and organs of the head, whereas longer waves, such as red and orange components, penetrate the tissues of the so-called "optical window." In the intact eye, effects of shorter, violet-to-blue light rays are very slight; green may be marked; and yellow, orange, and red increasingly stronger; but far red has very slight effect, and infrared none.

The demonstrated presence of porphyrins in the central nervous system of warm-blooded animals, the fact that administration of some porphyrin compounds demonstrably stimulates the onset of estrus, and the observation that porphyrin compounds absorb light in the red and blue-green regions, and emit red fluorescence when illuminated by whole light—all strongly suggest that one or more biochromes of this group must be actively involved in the photostimulation of mammalian and avian estrus.

Various porphyrin or porphyrinlike substances have been observed in materials generated by living organisms. An example is ambergris, the floating, waxy material disgorged from the stomach of the sperm whale. Following some preliminary Japanese observations, Lederer and Tixier extracted from a kilogram of ambergris 150 g of ether-insoluble residue from which they were able to recover some 30 mg of protoporphyrin and about 10 mg of mesoporphyrin. It has been suggested that the source of these discharged porphyrins may lie in the whale's heavy consumption of squid, whose hard, sharp beaks, remaining as indigestible residues, may lacerate the inner lining, inducing internal bleeding. Consequently, the hemoglobin introduced into the lumen may undergo degradation, whether due to the consumer's enzymes or via those of bacterial organisms, to afford protoporphyrin, part of which, in turn, may be reduced to mesoporphyrin.

Mesoporphyrin is characteristic in the feces of patients with porphyria and liver disorders, and fecal protoporphyrin has been found in cases of intestinal bleeding or consequent upon the ingestion of blood. Such observations lend credence to the suggested origin of the ambergris porphyrins.

Porphyrins as a chemical class occupy a remarkable position, not solely through the fact of their universal synthesis in organisms and their paramount role in vital metabolic processes, but also because of the high relative integrity of the cyclic tetrapyrrolic skeleton, once it has been synthesized. Of all biochemically synthesized organic molecular classes, the porphyrins, once discharged from the organism, whether through excretion or following death, are supreme in chemical stability, notably as regards the fundamental tetrapyrrolic ring itself. Some such compounds maintain their fundamental molecular characteristics through vast periods of time and despite wide variations in environmental conditions. Being spectroscopically identifiable and measurable, even minute traces of porphyrins may serve as useful biochemical fossils in samples failing to yield other chemicals diagnostic of biological origin. Thus, the relative concentrations and degree of chemical reduction of long-buried porphyrins serve as indicators of time, among other factors, and thus as rough indices of geological age.

Fossil porphyrins, notably several derived from chlorophyll degradation, have been encountered in ancient muds of freshwater and marine basins, e.g., greenish pigments in recent Black Sea sediments, in older deposits bearing mussel (*Mytilus*) fossils, in still earlier levels yielding *Dreissensia* and other Caspian molluscs of glacial times, and in argillaceous sediments near Sevastopol, belonging to the Tertiary period. Similarly characterized greenish, chlorophyllically derived porphyrin fossils have been found in other old marine and lake sediments; some of these exhibited evidence of having been long exposed to chemically reducing conditions.

The researches of Treibs, published as far back as the middle and earlier 1930s, contain reports of porphyrins in even far earlier deposits than any previously discussed, including bituminous rocks, coal, shale, asphalt, mineral waxes, and other ancient materials. He found, in essentially all deposits investigated, four chief porphyrin fractions, namely desoxyphylloerythrin and desoxyphylloerythroporphyrin, which he decided came from chlorophyll, and mesoporphyrin and mesoetioporphyrin, which he concluded had arisen from the decomposition of animal hemes. In most of the samples investigated by Treibs, the former pair of porphyrins excelled the latter two, often by 95 percent of the total porphyrins recovered.

The additional observation that these fossil porphyrins were present chiefly as bases, and only in minor part as mono- or dicarboxylic acids, led to the natural conclusion that both the degraded types of porphyrin, plant and animal, had been modified by slow, continued hydrogenation at the site.

Estimated quantities of total porphyrins in various petroleums varied from mere traces (0.004 to 0.020 mg) through medium amounts (0.5 to 2.0 mg) to fairly substantial concentrations (20 mg) per 100 g of the oil. One Trinidad oil specimen of Tertiary or Cretaceous origin yielded about 40 mg of porphyrins per 100 g.

Porphyrins recovered from very ancient Esthonian fire shale, constituted of Devonian, Silurian, even perhaps Cambrian deposits, thus represented ages of several hundred million years, and were preponderantly of the acid type, i.e., desoxyphyllerythrin, with but one propionic acid group, and mesoporphyrin, with two such side chains. A 50-g sample of such material yielded about 0.010 mg (10 μg) of porphyrins.

Porphyrins, accompanied by carotenoids, were readily recoverable in recent and older marine and lake sediments. Some of our own earlier researches as well as others pursued by E. F. Corcoran revealed phaeophytins a and b from the respective chlorophyll precursors, as characteristic of more recent deposits, while in older (deeper) strata these were converted to their corresponding phaeophorbides through hydrolytic cleavage of the phytol ester link. Corcoran's survey included sediments not only off the coast of Southern California, but areas yielding similar cores from the Mississippi Delta, Gulf of Mexico, and Acapulco region.

EPILOGUE

"You are old, Father William," the doctor declared,
"And your skin has porphyrial blight;
Your specimen's pink, and your body won't bear
Exposure to our solar light."

"Very true," he replied, "and it's surely no fun;
It's my liver and blood, don't you see?
They're resolved to create uroporphyrin I,
While I need uroporphyrin III."

BILINS OR BILICHROMES
(App., 60-64)

Among the more commonly occurring linear tetrapyrrolic pigments or bilichromes are the following:

Bilirubin (red-brown; orange-red in solution) $C_{33}H_{36}O_6N_4$
(App., 62)

Biliverdin (blue-green dehydrobilirubin) $C_{33}H_{34}O_6N_4$
(App., 61;
pls. 45, 47, 48)

Glaucobilin (blue or violet red crystals) $C_{33}H_{38}O_6N_4$
(App., 63)

Mesobiliviolin (carmine) $C_{33}H_{40}O_6N_4$

Mesobilirubin (orange) $C_{33}H_{40}O_6N_4$

Urobilin (brown-orange to yellow) $C_{33}H_{42}O_6N_4$

The list is led by a couple of prominent, characteristic end products of hemoporphyrin breakdown, encountered in urine, feces, and bile, the hepatic secretion in the gallbladder of man and other mammals. The golden-yellow, sometimes greenish or dark-brown colors of bile are indeed due to varying proportions of bilirubin and its oxidized (actually dehydrogenated) derivative, biliverdin, the latter being notably present especially in herbivorous mammals. These two bilichromes are degradation products of hemoglobin.

Human jaundice is triggered by occlusion of the bile duct, entailing increasing quantities of bile pigments entering the blood, hence to the pronounced yellowing of the skin. The responsible pigment in jaundiced skin is bilirubin, variously reported in older (chiefly medical) literature as biliphaein, bilifuscin, cholepyrrin, or haematoidin. It is dissolved in the bile fluid as a sodium salt, and may be found also in gallstones as an insoluble calcium bilirubinate.

In crystalline form, bilirubin is red-brown in color, insoluble in water or dilute acids, sparingly soluble in chloroform (more so when hot), diethyl ether, ethanol, carbon disulfide, or benzene. Its alkaline salts are orange-red in solution. Exhibiting no spectral absorption bands in the visible range, its solutions show merely increasing absorption toward the violet end. Its zinc chelate in ammoniacal solution, however, exhibits absorption bands in the red, yellow, and green spectral regions.

On mild oxidation, whether through metabolic processes or with hydrogen peroxide, or even on exposure of its aqueous alkaline solution to air, bilirubin is converted into biliverdin through the loss of two hydrogen atoms from the central region of the linear molecular chain (App., 61, 62).

Biliverdin is recoverable as a dark-green, amorphous solid mass or as dark-green plates or prisms with a violet surface glance. Like bilirubin, it is insoluble in water or dilute acids and dissolves only sparingly in methanol, ether, or chloroform. It is soluble in benzene, carbon disulfide, glacial acetic acid, or concentrated sulfuric acid, and in alkalis, wherein it forms salts of bright-green color, manifesting strong light absorption in the deep-red spectral regions.

Urobilin (stercobilin), a brownish pigment recoverable from chloroform or acetone in the form of yellow needles, is a product of the reduction of bilirubin by mammalian intestinal bacteria. Readily soluble in methanol, ethanol, pyridine, or glacial acetic acid, it is less so in acetone or chloroform, and insoluble in petroleum ether or carbon disulfide. Its amyl alcohol solution exhibits a green fluorescence, while in concentrated hydrochloric or sulfuric acid its solutions are red. It may be salted out from urine by saturation with ammonium sulfate and may subsequently be extracted from the slurry with alcohol. In such a solution, urobilin manifests a broad absorption band between 486 and 508 nm. If zinc chloride or its acetate be added to the neutral solution, an additional maximum occurs near 486 nm.

Both uteroverdin, a green bilichrome formed in hemorrhagic placental tissues of the dog, and oöcyan, a blue or blue-green pigment extractable from eggshells of some gulls and numerous other wild birds, have been identified with biliverdin.

Relatively high concentrations of bilirubin may occur in the blood plasma of the horse in amounts averaging some 1.6 mg/ 100 ml. This pigment thus is prominent in contributing the high yellow color to the plasma. Fasting reportedly evokes a considerable elevation in the horse's plasma bilirubin level, which regresses after feeding.

While the bilichromes are more commonly regarded as appearing consequent upon the breakdown of porphyrins such as hemoglobin, there is ground for viewing them on occasion in another role, participating in iron metabolism. In secondary anemia of humans and of dogs, the intravenous injection of iron salts together with bilirubin has promoted the synthesis of hemoglobin. Bilirubin likewise accelerates hemopoiesis in bled rabbits. Whether indeed bilirubin, a waste product from the degradation of heme porphyrins, may serve the role of a hormone in hemoglobin generation is a question calling for further study. Minor quantities of bilirubin, biliverdin, and perhaps choleglobin as well have been isolated from red blood cells.

Of interest to comparative biologists is the occurrence of bilichromic pigments in certain plants. Blue phycocyans and red phycoerythrins serve as photosynthetic pigments, accessory to chlorophyll, in red marine algae, which characteristically inhabit bottoms beneath deeper waters than most algae. An outstanding bilichromic example, universal in green plants, is phytochrome (App., 64), a blue compound present in minute quantities, and indispensable for the triggering of various periodic processes initiated by incident light.

Phytochrome occurs in two alternate forms, P_{660} and P_{730}, often referred to as P_r and P_{fr} respectively, designating red and far-red. The pair of phytochromes involve a balanced, alternative placement of but a pair of hydrogen atoms each of which travels reversibly between the respective molecular sites. This paired intermigration of H atoms involves the transposition of two respective pairs of double bonds, one pair situated in a pyrrole ring at either end of the linear molecule or, alternatively, chained onto each ring as vinyl or ethyl radicals (see App., 64).

Of the two phytochromic isomers (perhaps more properly called tautomers), the far-red operative P_{730} sets off germination and respiration in seeds of higher plants, and of spores in mosses and ferns, the blossoming of long-day plants (or inhibition thereof in short-day species), etiolation (growth in darkness, without development of chlorophyll), cuticle pigmentation, elaboration of anthocyanins (e.g., in red cabbage, turnips, and apples), and several other structural and functional responses.*

The P_{660} phytochrome form is able to reverse many physiological reactions evoked by P_{730}. Even very short-time incidence of light absorbed by the former can delay flowering in some short-day plants otherwise scheduled to bloom following earlier exposure to light of such wavelength that only the P_{730} phytochrome had been effectively involved.

Numerous species among the lower animals are known to store, and may display, bilichromic pigments. The peritoneal cells of the medicinal leech, following the ingestion of hemoglobin, have been observed to secrete greenish-yellow and brown bilins, recoverable in the animal's feces. Digestive glands of such crustaceans as the crayfish *Cambarus* likewise yield a green bilichrome; and *Octopus bimaculatus,* following a diet of horse liver, secretes into its hepatopancreas a green bilichrome, along with the greenish porphyrin type referred to earlier.

---

*This precise consideration prompted one of L-G's characteristic questions: "Why and how does it happen, on a fall day, that one tree will blush red all over, while its close neighbors of the same kind still are green, or maybe go yellow first?" My answer: "Yes."

Further among the molluscs we find bilichromic pigmentation in both living tissues and shells. The red epidermal color of the terrestrial slug *Arion rufus* and the orange pigment from the shell of the abalone *Haliotis rufescens* have been called rufine and rufescine respectively. Recent studies by Rüdiger and Chapman have identified the abalone pigment rufescine as haliotisrubin, recoverable from the shells of a dozen species of *Haliotis,* and demonstrably arising from the animal's consumption of red algae, which synthesize the related red bilin phycoerythrin. Dr. D. L. Leighton gave the author three small, entire abalone shells (*Haliotis rufescens*) (pl. 46), embedded within a block of clear transparent plastic material, and recording, through the serial pigmentation of the shell material, the respective animals' diets throughout a whole year of experimental feeding. One specimen that had received solely red algae during the entire period developed a pink to red-colored outer shell surface, while the other two, which had received red algae alternating with *Macrocystis,* a brown kelp, during successive months, now each displayed across the outer shell surfaces clearly marked six white and six pink-to-red bands. The original consumers had deposited into the newly developing shell, at the edge of the fleshy mantle, haliotisrubin as a complex calcium salt or chelate derived originally from the red algal pigment phycoerythrin.

Rüdiger and Chapman discovered yet another interesting bilichrome, haliotisviolin, a violet, diketo compound closely related to haliotisrubin, in nine of their twelve abalone species, but have not recognized the algal source of this second pigment. It may well be derived from the same original precursor.

A prominent marine slug of Southern California waters enjoys the same diet of red algae as do the abalones. This is *Aplysia californica,* the so-called sea hare, which derives a purple ink, aplysioviolin, from its dietary red-algal bilichrome, phycoerythrin; and stores the substance in a specialized ink gland, thence secreting it into an ink sac. When disturbed, the animal discharges the richly pigmented ink into the surrounding water (or upon a collector's hand). Specimens from which all ink had been "milked out," and which subsequently had been denied red algae, being sustained entirely on a diet of brown kelp, failed to generate any ink, discharging only a colorless secretion until resupplied with red algae. The ink fluid of *Aplysia* contains, beside the pigment, certain malodorous and persistent chemicals which render it demonstrably distasteful to predators.*

The aplysioviolin itself, however, hardly can be involved as a part of the defense mechanism. Most likely it is a fortuitously included waste product, discharged whether in daylight or darkness, and at any depth, if the animal is threatened by so much as the touch of a suspected predator.

Among other invertebrates we encounter the arrestingly conspicuous blue coral *Heliopora caerulea* (pl. 45), of Australian and West Indo-Pacific waters, whose pigment was earlier characterized as helioporobilin, it being recognized as belonging to the bilin class. Later research by Rüdiger et al. showed the pigment to be a calcium-bonded biliverdin IX_a. Nothing is known of the significance of biliverdin in the metabolism of the coral.

The conspicuously colored, venomous oceanic jellyfish *Physalia physalis,* or Portuguese man-of-war carries biliverdin and/or isomers thereof in its blue tissues, and perhaps other bilichromes in the pale lavender-blue float, the pink-tinged crest, and greenish and purplish shades of blue in the reproductive and feeding structures. The different colors supposedly are evoked by the bilichrome's conjugation with various kinds of protein.

Certain insects display a blue, water-soluble pigment (perhaps a conjugated protein complex) which, upon hydrolysis, yields a bilichromic pigment, pterobilin, which, although not identical with either biliverdin or glaucobilin, closely resembles these compounds in several ways. The pigment was recovered from wings of Lepidoptera such as *Pieris brassicae, P. rapae, P. napi, Gonepterix rhamni, Catopsilia rurina* and *C. statera.* A yield of 8 mg of pterobilin was reported from the extraction of 125 g of wings from 6,000 specimens of *Catopsilia rurina.*

M. Passama-Vuillaume has shown that biliverdin, conjugated with protein, is responsible for the green pigmentation of the praying mantis *Mantis religiosa,* and is present also in both albino and normal phases of the migratory locust *Locusta*

*And nauseating to any collectors; as L-G remarked, after having been commissioned to collect some ink in the field, "The ink is not worth the stink."

migratoria. Thermally and photically induced oxidation of the biliverdin component gives rise to yellow and brown products, which in turn become bonded to proteins in the locust, but which remain uncombined in the mantis, thus evoking in the latter a series of differently colored phenotypes.

Numerous fishes, especially among the Belonidae or needle-fishes and the Cottidae, that is, sculpins, exhibit the blue-green color of bilins (undoubtedly biliverdin in most instances) in bones and scales. Indeed, skin, muscle, digestive tract, and eggs of the sculpin *Pseudoblennius percoides* contain the same bluish bilichrome-protein complex. Yamaguchi and others report this, and also the presence of biliverdin, conjugated with protein, partly via a sulfhydryl bond, in the blue scales of the parrot-fish *Scarus gibbus.* Like the needlefishes *Belone belone* and *Strongylura exilis,* the green skeletal pigment in some tunas, mackerel, and skipjack, for example, *Katsuwonus pelamis,* is identical with or closely allied to biliverdin. In some instances the green bilichromic pigment appears also in the flesh of some specimens, which as a result are avoided by some fisherman or buyers unders an impression that the color denotes presence of a toxic substance. The green color portends nothing harmful, however, and indeed disappears on cooking. The flesh, moreover, is as tasty as expected.

The extensive occurrence of bilins, notably biliverdin, in the shell of many bird species' eggs (pls, 47, 48), was surveyed earlier in discussing also the even wider incidence of porphyrins there. Before the research upon which the survey by Kennedy and Vevers had been conducted, earlier attention had been given to the pigment recoverable from the dark-green eggshells of the Australian emu *Dromiceius novae hollandiae.* The green egg, shaped and of the size and color of an avocado, yielded principally biliverdin IX_a, accompanied by a lesser amount of a yellow compound convertible by oxidation into biliverdin, hence concluded to have been bilirubin. The cassowary *Casuarius galatea* of New Guinea deposits a beautiful egg about one-third or one-quarter the size of an average watermelon, and similarly shaped, a prolate spheroid (pl. 48). Its shell has light-green, raised, mottled markings over the whole surface. The pigment, here again, very probably is biliverdin. Areas of the shell surface scraped smooth with a blade reveal a pale-blue surface, still more suggestive of biliverdin, as bonded to calcium.

The comprehensive physiological status of bilins remains obscure. Where they appear as insoluble salts, notably of calcium, as in skeletal materials, they presumably are inert metabolically. Moreover, they seem never to achieve effective concentrations beyond mere traces, unless we reserve judgment regarding the bilichromoproteins, whose more obvious concentrations may portend metabolic usefulness. Their sources in eggshells and in the skeletons of some fishes reside manifestly in the heme. In invertebrate tissues and skeletal materials, the derivation of bilichrome pigments has to reside in the animals' universal propensity for synthesis of tetrapyrroles. The blue-green skin, fins, mouth parts, even mucus and other integumentary surfaces of numerous fishes (not to be confused with the cerulean blues of many species) often involve bilichromoproteins, which may be functional in the generation of mucopolysaccharides or glycoproteinaceous materials of mucus. We have at present no clue as to whether the tetrapyrroles may serve a role in the deposition of skeletal materials in those instances wherein such pigments occur.

8
Flavins, Purines, and Pterins

These three classes, relatively minor in respect to visibility in organisms, are placed in a common chapter, not only because the data regarding them are not columinous, and therefore would lead to a relatively short independent discussion of each, but, more importantly, because there are structural chemical affinities between them, although they are typified by different biochemical origins and roles.

FLAVINS
(App., 65)

The flavins, sometimes referred to as lyochromes, are not visually obvious, but occur in minor concentrations as pale-yellow, water-soluble, chemically heterocyclic compounds (i.e., with both N and C atoms within their ring conformations) in all plant and animal cells so far as we know. They are characterized by (1) their solubility in all aqueous media, and insolubility in most of the typical fat solvents; (2) yellow color in solution, turning to orange-red when crystalline; (3) manifestation of greenish-yellow fluorescence in neutral solution, which vanishes on substantial acidification or alkalization; and (4) relative stability toward mild oxidizing agents, yet (5) reversibly reduced to a colorless state by reducing agents such as $Na_2S_2O_4$ (hyposulfite). The colored solutions also display characteristic maxima of absorption and of fluorescent emission (see below).

Flavin materials were formerly denoted by various names in accordance with the source from which isolation had been made, for example, lactoflavin from milk whey, ovoflavin from egg albumin, cytoflav from hog's heart, renoflavin from kidney, uroflavin recoverable from urine, and so on. In most instances by far the product is the same compound, riboflavin, so named from its conjugant, ribityl alcohol, or more commonly, ribitol, from a pentose or 5-carbon sugar, ribose (App., 65). Riboflavin occurs in the aforementioned materials and in many other widely different biological substances. Like the carotenoids, it appears to be synthesized de novo only by plant cells, from which animals obtain it, directly or indirectly, through their nutrition. In green plants the highest concentrations of the flavin occur in the growing leaves. Flavins, notably riboflavin, occur in tissues either free or, more often, conjugated as flavoprotein. Flavopurines and phosphoflavins also have been detected in nature. A riboflavin-phosphoric acid-protein complex is the so-called yellow oxidation enzyme, and riboflavin itself is an important component of the vitamin B_2 complex.

Riboflavin's salient biochemical function as an oxidase, or oxidizing catalyst, rests upon its role as a reversible hydrogen acceptor. It occupies an indispensable link in a chain of cellular oxidation-reduction systems.

Since their concentrations and tinctorial powers are very low, flavins and their complexes are quite inconspicuous as actual pigments, save that certain animal tissues may reveal their flavin content by the yellow-green fluorescence evoked under u.v. light. Actual concentrations or yields are expressed usually in μg (often written alternatively as γ) signifying thousandths of a milligram, per gram, rather than as mg per 100 g. Three kg of fresh eggs have yielded a mere 15 mg; 5400 l of whey nearly 1 g; 10 to 20 mg of the flavin have been recovered from a kilogram of kidney or liver tissue. All of these are considered relatively rich sources of flavin among animal tissues or products.*

Riboflavin is crystallizable from alcohol as yellow-orange, stellate needles which show no melting point but decompose with charring at high temperatures between 274 and 293°C. Its neutral aqueous solutions show an absorption band in the violet

*For the optional interest of chemically oriented readers, the empirical formula of riboflavin is $C_{17}H_{20}O_6N_4$; its alternative chemical designation is 6,7-dimethyl-9-d-ribityl-benzisoalloxazine; its molecular weight, 376.36; and its supposed structural designation shown in the Appendix, no. 65.

at 445 nm, and three ultraviolet maxima, at 372, 269, and 225 nm. Aqueous solutions of riboflavin are fluorescent, but least so, whereas in pyridine the property is maximal.

The fluorescence of riboflavin in aqueous systems varies but little through a fairly wide range of pH values between 3 and 9, remaining substantially constant between 5.5 and 8.0, but diminishing sharply beyond the range in either direction, according to whether the solution be rendered slightly more acidic or a little more alkaline. The fluorescent band lies in the green region at ca. 562 to 565 nm, while in a crystalline state the compound exhibits increased fluorescence accompanied by an elevation to a higher wavelength—596 nm.

The flavin molecule exhibits no fluorescence when conjugated with protein. Flavoproteins show molecular weights ranging from 60,000 to nearly 80,000.

Reversible chemical reducibility is an important attribute of riboflavin, and can be rather spectacular in that it is demonstrable readily and easily in a test tube. If a small "knife-point" trace of sodium hyposulfite is introduced into the yellow, fluorescent aqueous solution, both color and fluorescence are quenched instantaneously on stirring by merely swirling the tube in the fingers. But the original appearance is then restored simply by shaking the system in air.

Riboflavin is further characterized by its resistance to heat, dilute acids, and various oxidizing agents, as well as by its ready degradation by alkalies and light. Its other chemical properties, as well as methods of recovering and isolating it, are discussed in *Animal Biochromes,* among other sources.

The actual concentrations of flavin in plants are not rich, but it is to be borne in mind that the primary synthesis of the compound apparently resides in the fresh leaves, where it is renewed continuously. Thus it develops that, while animals indeed excrete some of their ingested flavin, they may yet accumulate and store higher concentrations of it in certain organs than do plants, the original manufacturers. Red algae have been reported to store more flavin than do the greens and browns. Relatively high yields have been reported also from certain yeasts and bacteria.

Certain insects manifest high flavin concentrations, which,

moreover, exhibit increases with advancing age. Various species of marine cirripeds (barnacles) and isopods inhabiting well-oxygenated waters tend to store less flavin per gram of fresh tissue, for example, 1-2 μg/g, than other species living amphibiously or in otherwise less favorable respiratory conditions, which have yielded from 3 to 14 μg/g. Flavin is regarded as playing a role in melanin formation in some crabs, whose integumentary cells serving as precursors to melanophores contain riboflavin.

Among vertebrates, liver, kidney, and other glandular tissues are richest in flavin, which is conjugated with protein for the most part. Considerable quantities of flavin are voided in mammalian urine and feces. Human infants may pass from 22 to 207 μg of urinary flavin, while an adult may lose as much as 900 μg, in a 24-hour period. Urinary flavin losses cease sharply at the onset of B_2 avitaminosis in experimental animals such as rats.

Riboflavin, whether free or conjugated with protein, is a hydrogen-transporting agent in cellular and muscular metabolic processes, and thus is involved in the utilization of carbohydrates.

It has been suggested that the rich stores of flavin in the eyes of some fishes may facilitate more acute vision in diffuse light by transforming certain longer waves into yellow-green radiations residing within the range of maximal optical activity. There remains also the fact of flavin and flavoprotein residing in the skin of numerous fishes, notably in close association with melanin aggregates, as was evident in certain crabs as well.

Both flavins and carotenoids may serve important physiological functions not yet understood in some bivalved molluscs. For example, concentrations of carotenoids, flavin, and ascorbic acid (vitamin C) have been found to be considerably higher in the metabolically active visceral mass than in gills, mantle, and other tissues of both oyster (*Ostrea edulis*) and another lamellibranch, *Gryphia angulata*.

The eggs of several elasmobranch fish species undergo a diminution in flavin content following fertilization. Examples are the sharks *Mustelus vulgaris* and *Scilliorhinus canalicula,* whose ovarian eggs, showing 11.5 and 4.6 μg/g respectively, lose 52 and 37 percent of their respective flavin concentrations after fertilization, while the ova of the skate *Raja asteria* lose 39 per-of their flavins when fertilized. The developing embryo of the shark *Carcharinus commersonii,* however, was diminished only slightly in flavin concentration compared with that of the egg. But the *total* quantity of flavin underwent a considerable increase, due to the storage and supply of flavin in the animal's yolk sac. That organ in another shark, *Squalus blainvilii,* possesses flavin concentrations as high as 3.2 μg/g, while the animal's embryo shows flavin levels less than half this value. This elevation of flavin levels in fishes' bodies is rather general. The developing stages and adults of the freshwater eel, *Anguilla vulgaris,* provide useful examples. Larval stages weighing but 0.39 g yield low concentrations of flavin, for example, about 1.8 μg/ g; yellow juveniles of fourfold the weight carry double the flavin concentrations, whereas adult males (115 g) manifest threefold such concentrations, corresponding respectively to an 8-fold and 900-fold augmentation of the larval flavin supply. The growing eels would appear to be efficient assimilators of dietary flavin useful in their growth metabolism.

While blood and muscle of adult female eels carry but small quantities of flavin, and spleen, gills, heart, and kidney contain but slightly more, the ovary and liver are appreciably richer (5.3-10 μg/g), and dorsal skin the richest of all tissues, 12-26 μg/g; indeed, skin from the back of adult males may attain flavin concentrations as high as 37 μg/g. Flank skin yields considerably less, and white, ventral integument only bare traces.

Flavin in the eel's skin is conjugated with protein and is localized in the pigmented layer bearing carotenoids and melanophores, but lacking in guanine-rich areas, as in the shiny-white belly skin. Similar contrasts apply to flavin in the scales of carp. It appears more than likely that riboflavin may play a role in controlling photostimulated generation of melanin within the specialized cells.

Fish species which lack scales or possess only minute, concealed scales tend to store considerably more flavin in the skin, whereas scaly fishes often possess instead a blue, fluorescent compound, first called fluorescyanin, and later identified as a pterin pigment, ichthyopterin. The correlation between flavin richness and locus of melanophores in basal epidermal strata holds for the eel (*Anguilla vulgaris*), conger (*Conger vulgaris*), blennies such as *Blennius gattorugine* and *Muroena helena,* and the lamprey *Petromyzon marinus.*

It has been observed that similar relationships seem to apply to crustaceans. The hypoderm, or thin layer of integument immediately beneath the shell of a dozen or more species of crab whose tissues bear rich melanin supplies, also yields appreciable quantities of riboflavin. This condition does not hold for allied species which lack the dark pigment. Variations have been noted in hypodermal riboflavin concentrations during the molting cycle. Some residual flavin may be encountered in the cast skeleton. The reduced quantities of hypodermal flavin characteristic of freshly molted individuals are augmented as normal feeding is resumed.

The blood plasma of certain Brazilian snakes has been investigated for both riboflavin and carotenoids. Riboflavin amounting to as much as 200 μg/100 ml has been reported from a poisonous species, *Bothrops jararaca,* and from the nonvenomous *Eudryas bifossatus.* Neither of these yielded detectable plasma carotenoids, whereas plasma from the rattlesnake *Crotalus terrificus,* and from *Xenodon merremii* yielded xanthophylls but not carotene or significant amounts of flavin.

PURINES
(App., 66-67)

This group of compounds, being in fact without color, hardly are to be classed among the biochromes proper. They will receive brief consideration here, however, since certain members of the series, notably guanine and uric acid, effect an opaque whiteness, sometimes with glistening, silvery aspects, or even iridescent colors of interference, notably among some of the lower animals.

The naturally occurring purines of special zoological significance are simple hydroxy and amino derivatives of the fundamental purine ring, not itself occurring simply as such in the living world. The hydroxypurines xanthine and hypoxanthine are to be found in tissues and body fluids of animals. Uric acid, a trioxypurine (actually also a tribasic acid due to tautomerism, i.e., involving alternative placement of H atoms between positions on N atoms of the ring and on keto side chains, as shown in App., 67), is a degradation product of purines in many phyla, but also constitutes the chief nitrogenous waste product of protein metabolism in birds and terrestrial reptiles, which void it in solid form with their feces. This widely occurring purine is also a normal excretory product in the urine of mammals, and in the metabolic wastes of the sea anemone *Metridium senile,* which voids the material in a yellowish ring of slime, surrounding the circle of tentacles and settling down about the pedal disc.

Xanthine, uric acid, and other purines accompany pterins in the wings of many butterflies and moths. Uric acid, a catabolyte from the chrysalid stage, is deposited as part of the overall pattern in the wings of the adult butterfly. Some degree of sexual dichromatism is thus expressed, males excelling females by ratios of about 5:3 in their wing uric acid content.

The monoaminopurines adenine and guanine (App., 66a, b) are components of the vitally important nucleic acids and nucleosides of cells. Such purine derivatives arise in part from the dietary nucleoproteins, although some animals undoubtedly synthesize them, most likely from the amino acids arginine and histidine.

There are extensive reviews (e.g., those cited in *Animal Biochromes*) of protein and purine metabolism in the animal phyla. There seems to have been an increasing tendency for animals to generate enzymes capable of breaking down purine compounds. The vertebrates, unlike most invertebrate forms, possess enzymes which deaminate, or liberate ammonia from, the nucleosides adenosine and guanosine.

Among the purines that constitute the white or silvery areas of integumentary structures, guanine is the greatly outstanding example, while uric acid is observed in some instances. A remarkable correlation is evident, notably among certain reptiles, amphibians, insects, and—suspectedly—some molluscs between purine metabolism and coloration patterns at mating season. It has been suggested that, since much of this coloration and/or pattern modification is correlated with altered and accelerated nucleoprotein metabolism at the very time of spermatogenesis, there must be simultaneous elaboration *and* degradation of nucleins, whence the consequent presence of excess purine residues, leading to their increased deposition in exposed areas.

Earlier reference was made to the highly specular, blue-reflective deposits of crystalline guanine in the eyes of many deep-sea fishes and in certain reptiles, notably crocodilians, leading to the expression of nocturnal eyeshine, and believed to serve usefully in augmenting vision through dimly lighted regions.

The white or iridescent so-called leucophores in the skins of fishes, amphibians, some lizards and cephalopods, often referred to alternatively as iridocytes or guanophores, owe their physically reflective properties to microcrystalline deposits of guanine (App., 66b). The silvery lateral lines of many fishes and the stratum arginatum in white layers of their ventral skin are especially rich in guanine. Excretory cells in the blood of numerous sea squirts (ascidians or tunicates) are laden with such purines as xanthine, guanine, or uric acid (App., 67), which impart a generally white aspect to such materials. The guanophores of some fishes may become so gorged with the white or iridescent, sharp platelets or otherwise crystalline guanine as to rupture the cell walls, releasing the crystals into intercellular spaces, where they remain chemically inert.

PTERINS
(App., 68-70)

For interested readers, a glance at the respective structural formulas of riboflavin, purines such as guanine, and pterins, for example, xanthopterin, will readily illustrate the fundamental chemical relationships between these three types; each involves the fundamental pyrimidine ring. The pterins carry also the 6-membered pyrazine ring, condensed to the pyrimidine cycle at the 5-6 carbon positions. Here they differ from the flavin molecule in that the latter bears yet a third ring, that is, a 6-carbon benzoid structure, condensed to the *opposite* (2-3) pair of carbons in the pyrazine moiety. The purines, representing the smallest and simplest of the three classes, bears a 5-atom imidazole ring condensed to the 5-6 carbons of its pyrimidine nucleus, in place of the pyrazine cycle carried there by the pterins.

A. E. Needham's recent book, *The Significance of Zoochromes* (1974), lists more than a score of known pterins, showing colors ranging from white (i.e., *none*) through pale yellow, yellow, orange, to red, and the solution of each manifesting one or more absorption maxima in ultraviolet and/or visible spectra; moreover, most of the pterins are fluorescent.

Members of the pterin group, because of their chemical and metabolic alliance with the purines, formerly were included among these. And we have noted that they bear also close chemical and physiological kinships with the flavins, which might have justified their earlier inclusion in that category. The name *pterin* (from the Greek *pteron*, "wing") derives from an earlier term "lepidopterin," referring to the fact that these nitrogenous, heterocyclic breakdown products are incident prominently in the wings of butterflies (*Lepidoptera*, "scaly wings"), wherein they confer not only whiteness, as do the purines, but, unlike the latter, frequently yellow, orange, and red areas as well.

Of the naturally occurring animal pigments, the carotenoids, hemes and porphyrins, bilins, melanins, riboflavin, and even the quinones and ommochromes have been recognnized in more organismal sites, for example, from ten for the ommochromes, to thirty-six for hemes and porphyrins, than have members of the pterin class, which are reported in only about a half-dozen sites, viz., epidermis, sense organs, vertebrate neural crest, testis sheath of arthropods, gut wall, and urine (as waste). Moreover their concentrations are extremely low at all sites (see below). Among functions served by pterins and their derivatives, it is likely that they constitute biochemical reductants, acting at respiratory substrate horizons, and perhaps early in the photoactivation stages of photosynthesis.

Characterized by a nitrogen content of 30 to 40 percent, the pterins are relatively polar compounds, fairly water-soluble in most instances, and insoluble in the common organic solvents. Possessing an amphoteric character, they are dissolved more readily in dilute acids or alkalies than in neutral aqueous systems. Some, but not all of the pterins respond as do the purines to the murexide test, wherein evaporative oxidation with concentrated nitric acid on a steam bath, followed by alkalization of the dry residue yields violet- to blue-violet-colored salts of purpuric acid. Certain pterins are recoverable in good crystalline form, while others may be obtained only as microcrystals or as crystalline derivatives of other compounds. Melting points are but poorly definable, these compounds tending merely to decompose at high temperatures. Thus chemical identification is difficult, and diagnosis must rely upon nitrogen content, absorption spectra, fluorescent and adsorptive characters.

Contrasting with flavins, pterins are sensitive to oxidation with permanganate in acetic acid media, with accompanying quenching of fluorescence. Like flavins, however, pterins are reducible to nonfluorescing, colorless derivatives by hyposulfite, this effect being reversible by shaking in air. This property is reminiscent of riboflavin's physiologically vital role as a cellular oxidation-reduction catalyst, and suggests the possibility of a parallel role fulfilled by pterins. Indeed certain pterins may serve as coenzymes analogous to the flavoproteins (see below).

The occurrence of pterins is in such minute concentration that huge quantities of raw source materials must be processed in order to yield enough of the refined product for reliable study. Thus sufficient xanthopterin had to be harvested from 250,000 butterfly wings; for urothion, 1,000 l of urine; and for ichthyopterin 25 kg of carp scales. Examples could be multiplied.

Glandular and hypodermal tissues of crustaceans are equally scanty in total pterin content, and offer additional problems in that much extraneous tissues must first be dispensed with. Raw materials, first extracted of all lipids with acetone or ether, are treated with certain alcohols, dilute acetic acid, or dilute alkali. Pterins thus recovered are resolved by fractional precipitational procedures, followed by reprecipitation or by chromatographic adsorption and subsequent individual elution from the separated zones of now-colored powdery sorbent.

A few commoner and better-known pterin compounds, and the insects that bear them, are the following:

Lepidopterans	*Pterins*
Pieris brassicae, P. napi	Leucopterin (white) App., 69
Gonepteryx rhamni	Leucopterin Guanopterin (white) Xanthopterin (yellow) App., 68 Erythropterin (orange to red) Mesopterin (white)
Catopsilia rurina	Xanthopterin, chrysopterin
Appia nero, Catopsilia argante, Colias edusa, Euchloe cardamines	Xanthoptrin, erythropterin, guanopterin, leucopterin
Hymenoptera (wasps; hornets)	
Vespa crabro, V. germanica, V. vulgaris	Xanthopterin, leucopterin, mesopterin

The white pterin leucopterin, which responds to the murexide test, was for that reason earlier confused with uric acid. Extracted from the detached, dried wings of pierid butterflies with ammonium hydroxide, the compound is recovered accordingly as its ammonium salt. Wings from about 215,000 *Pieris* specimens, aggregating 1164 g in weight, yielded 31.9 g of crude lepidopterin, corresponding to some 0.1 mg per wing specimen.

Guanopterin's properties resemble those of guanine. It yields fine, colorless, needlelike crystals and provides a highly crystallizable sulfate which is only slightly water soluble.

Xanthopterin is recovered often as an insoluble barium salt. The liberated pterin exhibits bands at 391, 360, 267, and 243 nm. In glacial acetic acid solution it manifests two faint bands at 390 and 330 nm, and a strong maximum at 280 nm. Thus the whole spectral display takes place in the shortwave, ultraviolet region. The compound responds positively to the murexide test. Its fluorescent behavior is additive to these spectral data in facilitating its identification; it fluoresces with a yellow color in weak acid, clear blue in neutral aqueous media, and blue-green in alkali. Its adsorptive behavior and fluorescence in the adsorbed state are also typical. From mildly acidified methanol, for example, xanthopterin is very firmly adsorbed upon powdered alumina as a yellowish zone, affording intense yellow-green fluorescence in u.v. light.

Air-dried wings from 250 male *Gonepteryx rhamnus* aggregated a weight of only 7.4 g. Following removal of lipids by ether extraction, treatment with ammonia yielded 0.65 mg of xanthopterin per insect. This is the same pterin that imparts the yellow integumentary colors to the bodies of wasps and hornets.

Several Japanese researches have revealed xanthopterin as contributing the yellow color to the epidermis of the larval, lemon-colored mutant of the silk moth *Bombyx mori*. Uric acid, as well as white, crystallizable pterins, occur there also, but in larger proportions than in the skin of the white mutant (see *Animal Biochromes*).

The wide distribution of pterins in the above and allied Hymenoptera has been explored by Leclercq, who employed a modification of Ford's murexide test by exposure of suspected specimens to free chlorine, followed by treatment with ammonia, thus affording a brilliant purple color in the presence of the pterin.

Hymenoptera of the Northern Hemisphere were observed often to display large yellow spots of the pterin compound, whereas inhabitants chiefly characteristic of the Southern Hemisphere and tropical climes seemed often apt to lack such markings. Among the aculeate or stinging types, genera showing a strongly petiolated primary abdominal segment usually lack yellow spots; Vespidae (wasps such as yellow jackets) and Sphecidae (thread-waisted wasps) with bright yellow marking were commonly referable to forms possessing sessile first abdominal segments.

Mesopterin exhibits the appearance, solubility characteristics, chemical makeup, and feeble alkalinity all suggestive of a position intermediate between leucopterin and xanthopterin.

Erythropterin, the darkest colored of all common members of the class, is met with in the red parts of pierids' wings, for example, *Appia nero* and *Euchloe cardamines.* Orange-pigmented areas in the wings of male *Cotopsilia argante* and *Colias edusa* bear mixtures of erythropterin and xanthopterin.

Erythropterin is recovered by ammoniacal extraction of the raw sources, followed by reprecipitation with hydrochloric acid. It is very water soluble, its solution manifesting a bright, intense red color and spectral absorption maxima at 450, 420, and 300 nm. Its nitrogen content is lower than that of most pterins; it shows fluorescence in dilute acetic acid, and adheres more firmly to adsorbent powders than does xanthopterin. Both of these pterins are reducible to colorless derivatives by treatment with zinc dust and formic acid, affording nascent hydrogen.

Chrysopterin [Gk. *chrysopteros*, "golden-winged"], an acidic, yellow pterin, is characterized by qualities somewhat intermediate between those of xanthopterin and erythropterin. Like the latter, it exhibits violet-blue fluorescence in dilute acids; more reminiscent of xanthopterin, it is strongly adsorbed by alumina, and therein manifests a green-yellow fluorescence. Its barium salt is brown-yellow, amorphous, and more soluble than the corresponding xanthopterin salt.

Red and yellow eye-colors of the fruit-fly *Drosophila melanogaster* are believed to involve pterin pigments. One such compound which has been isolated, called drosopterin, shows a darker-red color than erythropterin, and an absorption maximum at 465 nm in water.

Certain green-colored insects, including orthopterous hunting or plant-devouring species, are believed to owe their colors to the presence of a blue bilichromoprotein, plus a yellow, water-soluble nonprotein compound. The green hemolymph contains the same two pigments, while the yellow member is found also in the hypoderm. The pentatomid bugs *Nezara viridula, N. viridula torquata,* and *Palomena viridissima,* which subsist upon the fruit and leaves of various plants, have very green wings, the color again arising from the presence of blue and yellow components. The yellow pigment is granular and is chiefly xanthopterin, while the blue fraction more than likely is a bilichromoprotein, as in other instances.

Lampyrine is a red-fluorescing, pterin-like pigment in tissues of several lampyrid beetles. This rose-red compound, incident in the pronotal zone of *Photinus marginellus,* renders the beetle fluorescent in the rose-red spectral region as viewed through a fluorescent microscope. It is disposed as minute, birefringent spherites of some 7×10^{-4} to 3×10^{-3} mm in diameter, chiefly in the male gonad, but also in adipose tissue under the pronotum and subcutaneously in thorax and abdomen. The pigment is very stable when stored in a dry condition, and was first encountered in specimens from a collection made sixty years earlier. It is soluble in acids and bases, but not in neutral aqueous systems, nor in the various typical organic solvents.

In acidic solution, lampyrine manifests a rose color, an absorption maximum at 565 nm, and bright-orange fluorescence. In strong alkali, the compound is of a dull-blue color, and the fiery red fluorescence exhibits a maximum at 650 nm. These alkaline solutions fade to yellow-green in color on irradiation. Oxidation with nitric acid destroys both color and fluorescence as displayed by lampyrine in acidic solutions. A melting point of 315°C was determined on a sample of the refined material. The compound reportedly does not respond to the murexide test, nor to Ehrlich's diazo reagent, aqueous ferric chloride, or zinc and hydrochloric acid. Therefore the classification of laympyrine as indeed a pterin has been questioned. It seems to characterize most lampyrid beetles examined, but not some closely related orders.

A pterin is believed to be responsible for fluorescence of materials in crustacean hypoderm, for example, that of the crab *Cancer pagurus*. It has been likened to xanthopterin, while the hepatopancreas appears to contain a different member of the series.

Pterins occur also in mammalian liver, feces, and urine, as well as in alfalfa, hay, and other plants. Whereas pterins appear to be excretory products, as laid down in considerable quantities by insect chrysalids during metamorphosis, none of these compounds appears in the excreta of the adult insects. Instead, they are manifest as bodily pigments, while uric acid is the catabolyte excreted.

During the late post-diapause of the developing eggs of the grasshopper *Melanoplus differentialis* there occurs a gradual diminution in riboflavin and an increasing genesis of pterinlike compounds, continuing during subsequent stages.

Xanthopterin exercises an inhibiting effect on melanin formation in vitro, while riboflavin has the opposite general effect.

It has been assumed that xanthopterin, oxidized to leucopterin, thus inhibits the tyrosine-tyrosinase reaction in the final stages.

The presence of xanthopterin in human urine ("uropterin") at dilutions of perhaps one part per million, hardly may contribute significantly to the characteristic yellow color, which is doubtless due chiefly to urochrome, a regular component related to the melanins.

Xanthopterin has been assigned as most probably the identity of the blue-fluorescent material in the eyes of numerous species of crustaceans, fishes, amphibians, and in the alligator. Indeed the choroid layer in the dogfish *Squalus acanthias,* and both retinal and choroid tissues in *Alligator mississippiensis* yield the blue-fluorescing material. No specific visual function has, however, been assigned to the pterin.

Ichthyopterin (App., 70), which characterizes the fluorescent scales of numerous fishes, and which behaves somewhat like aneurin (= thiamin or vitamin B_1), accelerates O_2 consumption in the rat brain during riboflavin deficiency. The O_2 consumption of pterin-bearing systems indeed is stimulated by photic energy; this may be important in visual processes, although no specific role has been assignable.

Biopterin is reputed to activate sexual processes in aphids, and is believed to help determine, through its relatively high concentrations in royal jelly, the development of the embryo as a queen bee instead of merely a neutral worker. A correlation has been observed between the eye-pterin content, endocrine organs, and the photoperiodic influence upon reproduction.

Pterins are recognized as affecting several aspects of development, such as stimulating cell proliferation in protozoans. Xanthopterin, while strongly stimulative of normal cell division, opposes the proliferation of tumorous growths.

These compounds also have been shown to possess antianemic properties, xanthopterin having been applied for the cure or prevention of anemia in young rats, monkeys, and young salmon. The same compound seems also to deter tumor growth in mice, whereas leucopterin, bearing but one more oxygen atom per molecule, failed in such a role, seeming indeed to counteract the effects of xanthopterin.

Ichthyopterin, the blue-fluorescing pterin encountered in

scales of fishes, exists in nature as a chromoprotein. The free compound $C_9H_{11}O_4N_6$ is recoverable from hot-water extracts as spherical bundles of pale-yellow needles. The compound is insoluble in water-immiscible solvents, but somewhat soluble in water, in ethanol at 60°, and in methanol or pyridine. In aqueous systems its fluorescence, evoked by u.v. light, exhibits a maximum at about 432 nm, and is most intense within a pH range between 5 and 8.

Ichthyopterin is thermostable, and is not broken down on exposure to the u.v. spectrum. It adheres readily to various sorptive powders, gives typical pterin reactions and, like xanthopterin, is reversibly reduced by hydriodic acid. It is reversibly reduced also by dithionite (= hydrosulfite or hyposulfite), to a colorless, nonfluorescent form. Its reduction by this reagent occurs less readily than does that of riboflavin; moreover, it is the more easily reoxidized by atmospheric oxygen. The compound may well serve in situ as a metabolic hydrogen transporter.

The more richly pigmented dorsal scales of goldfish or other carp species contain more ichthyopterin than the pale ventral scales, and consume about one-third more oxygen per hour. This O_2 consumption occurs, moreover, at the highest levels of pterin-rich parts than elsewhere in such scales.

Further physiological comparisons with vitamins B_1 and B_2 are evident in that vitamin-deficient rats or pigeons receiving ichthyopterin or certain other pterins recovered their growth rate, remained immune from the polyneuritis syndrome, recovered normal nerve excitability, body temperature, and glycogen reserves, and corrected bradycardia.

Ichthyopterin and thiamin are comparable as to restoration of the growth curve and normal chronaxie (nerve excitation), whereas certain synthetic pterins such as isoxanthopterin, as well as various carboxylic, hydroxy, and other chemical derivatives of active pterins were required in quantities five to ten-fold greater to produce comparable results.

Vitamin B_1 and B_2 deficiencies, induced simultaneously in experimental animals, for example, rats or pigeons, were negated by feeding or injecting ichthyopterin, leucopterin, or certain synthetic pterins.

9

Some Other Nitrogenous, Metal-Bearing Biochromes

Blut ist ein ganz besondrer Saft
—Mephisto, in Goethe's *Faust*

Here's metal more attractive.
Hamlet 3, 2

With Mephisto's declaration that blood is a juice of rarest quality, we must indeed agree, and with the further qualification that we are here moreover referring of necessity to bloods or body fluids of widely different species. Such fluids may display very different appearances in various organisms, for example, whether colorless, or shades of red, blue, green, yellow, or perhaps changing with oxygenation, all as partly suggested in the short rhymes introducing the earlier chapters dealing with carotenoids and with tetrapyrroles.

The intent in this concluding chapter is to consider a few of the more prominent and better-known examples of colored nitrogenous bodies encountered in the fluids and tissues of animals, notably such molecules as involve metallic ions in one state or another, that is, in addition to the outstanding iron-bearing example of hemoglobin, discussed in an earlier chapter.

Needham (1974) provides a list exceeding two pages (74-76) of more than two-score miscellaneous pigmentary substances distributed through the animal phyla, concerning which the exact chemical structure, and in many cases the physiological significance, remain unknown. Only a few examples will be selected from that list for further consideration here.

We shall deal in summary fashion with two respiratory

metalloprotein classes, namely hemocyanins and hemerythrins, as well as a few exceptional pigments of incompletely recognized function, including vanadochrome and related examples of limited distribution. The extraordinary cyanocobalamine vitamin B_{12}, a cobaltic tetrapyrrole complex, yet not actually a porphyrin, could as logically have been included in this chapter as in the site of its earlier treatment, the porphyrin section.

COPPER PROTEINS

Under this heading belong a large number of naturally occurring complexes, all affording oxidative-reductive functions of one kind or another, but of widely specific types. Indeed copper proteins occur widely distributed in tissues of diversified phyla. Naturalists will be most aware of the hemocyanins under this classification, since these occur in the most conspicuous concentrations in the circulatory fluids of several classes within the molluscs and arthropods, where they serve as oxygen carriers.

Under the appropriate section in his book (p. 49), Needham presents an informative, summarizing tabulation of the kinds, sources and various properties of naturally occurring copper proteins. A portion of his survey may be summarized in condensed form as shown on page 190.

The widely distributed incidence of protein-bound copper in living tissues is rather remarkable, and of recognized significance in certain cases. Most of these complexes are believed to involve the divalent or cupric (Cu^{2+}) state of copper; this is extensively typical of the several enzymes named, save for tyrosinase where the colorless monovalent cuprous Cu^+ ion is the one involved. In ceruloplasmin the ratio of Cu_2^+/Cu^+ is 1/1, and in oxyhemocyanins, the oxygen-carrying cuprotein type, the precise status of the copper ion has not been determined with finality. Certainly in the colorless reduced or deoxygenated condition of HCy, the Cu^+ state is the one present. But the oxygenated $HCyO_2$, blue in color, gives much evidence of involving both mono- and di-valent copper.

Aside from the O_2-carrying power of HCy, and the enzymic cuproproteins of specific function (e.g., tyrosinase, which

Protein	Source	Mol. Wt. (in 10^4 daltons)	Av. % Cu (No. Cu ions/mol.)	Color	Spectral λ max, nm
Oxyhemocyanin	Arthropods	40-100	0.17 (20)	blue	570
Oxyhemocyanin	Molluscs	200-900	0.245 (200-400)	blue	570
Ceruloplasmin	Mammalian serum	16	0.34 (8)	blue	610
Erythrocuprein	Mammalian erythrocytes	3.35	0.38 (2)	blue-green	655
Hepatocuprein	Mammalian liver	3.5	0.35 (2)	blue-green	660
Cerebrocuprein	Mammalian brain	3.5	0.30 (2)	blue-green	660
Lactocuprein	Milk	?	0.19 (?)	?	?
Dopamine β-hydroxylactase	Mammalian adrenals	29	0.50	colorless	——
Amine oxidases	Mammalian liver-mitochondria	25	0.075 (4)	colorless to pink	480
Uricase	Mammalian liver and kidney	12	0.06 (1)	?	?
Tyrosinase	Fungi	13	0.20 (4)	colorless	——

catalyzes the oxidation of tyrosine to afford ultimately dark melanin), most of these complexes remain of undefined role. But ceruloplasmin, the blue cuproprotein dissolved in minute traces in animal blood plasma, and which probably involves Cu^{2+} ions, is vitally important; its deficiency evokes serious pathological conditions. It catalyzes the oxidation of Fe^{2+} to Fe^{3+} iron, and hence may account in part for the long-recognized and vitally important need for copper in hemoglobin synthesis. Erythrocuprein, the copper protein occurring in traces within the red cells, may contribute to the fulfillment of a similar function.

Hemocyanin, the longest and best-known member of the copper proteins, is readily recognized in the shed blood of cephalopods, gastropods, and amphineurans or chitons, and is suspectedly present also in the body fluids of some bivalve molluscs. It occurs likewise in decapod, stomatopod, isopod, and amphipod malacostracan crustaceans, including the larger forms such as lobsters, crabs, prawns, etc., as well as the smaller classes. Other members of the arthropod phylum which carry hemocyanins are arachnoids, such as the king or horseshoe "crab" *Limulus polyphemus,* and arachnids, including some spiders and scorpions. No insects, however, have been reported to bear hemocyanin.

When one has occasion to dissect an octopus or an abalone (whether for study in the laboratory or for culinary purposes in the kitchen), the rather limpid, watery body fluid which spills out is colorless and slightly cloudy. But within minutes following exposure to atmospheric oxygen, it acquires a blue tint which readily deepens to a beautiful cerulean color. If dealing with a large crab or lobster, one may encounter, particularly during the animal's reproductive season, a carotenoid-red blood pouring from the opened blood vessels and sinuses. But this soon changes as the blue oxyhemocyanin is formed in air, and thus affords, jointly with the red astaxanthin, a resultant striking purple color.

If a sample of such blood, say molluscan, be allowed to stand, it clots to give a blue gel. If however, the freshly drawn blood is rapidly stirred, or is beaten with a whisk, thus defibrinating it, the clear blue fluid now bears little protein other than the hemocyanin, which may vary considerably in concentration according to species and other factors.

Chemical analyses of hemocyanins from different species have yielded such average values as the following for chemical composition: C: 53%, H: nearly 7%, N: about 16%, S: 1%, and O: roughly 23% by difference. The copper content varies from approximately 0.17 in arthropods to nearly 0.25 percent in molluscs, and the molecular weights of hemocyanins may vary widely among various species, as we have seen, being characterized by units of 10^5 among most arthropods, and reaching multiples of 10^6 within the molluscan phylum. *Limulus* HCy has been assigned a value close to 1,300,000, *Octopus,* 2,000,000, and *Helix,* the terrestrial snail, up to 5,000,000. In some species, such as *Helix* and *Octopus,* two forms of hemocyanin occur. *Octopus* possesses one type with molecular weight as reported above, and has a second, smaller grade as well. The diameters of the colloidal micelles, or macromolecules, of hemocyanin may likewise vary widely; those of the squid *Loligo*'s hemocyanin show an average diameter of 8 mμ, and of *Limulus,* twice as large, or 17 mμ.

Hemocyanin combines with oxygen in the ratio of 2 Cu/O_2. It unites also with cyanide, as does hemoglobin, and thus gives cyanhemocyanin, $RCu_2(CN)_4$, where R represents the relatively huge protein moiety. Hemocyanin's binding of carbon monoxide, however, reflects but about one-twentieth the affinity of hemoglobin therewith. The effect of hydrogen sulfide is to degrade hemocyanin.

Little yet is apparently known of the manner or loci in which hemocyanin synthesis occurs, but some concentration of copper has been observed in the crustacean hepatopancreas, wherein amounts of the stored ion may vary inversely with the blood-levels of hemocyanin. Blood hemocyanin and hepatopancreatic copper have been observed to decline in concentration following the molt of the European spider crab *Maja squinado,* and then to increase steadily as the new exoskeleton is forming and hardening. Observations parallel to these have been reported to follow experimental blood-letting in certain other crab species.

The midpoint of the single, broad, visible absorption maximum of oxyhemocyanins varies to some degree among different species, for example, the squid *Loligo,* the marine snail *Busycon,* the lobster *Homarus,* and the arachnoid *Limulus.* Still it commonly resides within the range between 570 and 581, and the shape of the overall absorption curve is closely similar among the species. The midpoint is, of course, more sharply defined once the colorless, light-scattering, colloidal fibrin has been eliminated from the solution.

Hemocyanins in general possess only about one-fourth the oxygen-combining capacity of hemoglobins. Considerable differences exist in this respect among species; there are, however, interesting correlations between habitat and activity of animals and the oxygen pressures needed for the full saturation of their blood. As instances, *Limulus* and certain bottom-dwelling gastropods possess hemocyanins saturable with oxygen at relatively low partial pressures of the gas. Such species are equipped for living under relatively limited conditions of aeration, but their general vitality is lowered and their activities curtailed by the low levels of dissolved oxygen available for respiration, via $HCyO_2 \longrightarrow HCy + O_2$ in their blood and tissues. Squid hemocyanin, on the contrary, is reversibly oxygenated only at high oxygen tensions; thus the squid is markedly sensitive to poorly aerated environmental conditions, but is very fleet and active in well-ventilated sites. Crustaceans are generally characterized by a somewhat intermediate physiological status, for whereas their hemocyanin resembles that of the squid in being readily oxygenated in generously aerated water, their concentrations of the copper protein are too low to afford prolonged vigorous activity. They accordingly are very susceptible to asphyxiation.

In numerous instances, hemocyanins serve not only as transporters of oxygen for respiratory needs but actually as a kind of storage bank, notably in species which reside for protracted intervals in oxygen-poor sites, exemplified by watery mud on the floor of their deep burrows.

Being globular proteins, the hemocyanins are well adapted for smooth circulation within the blood vessels, due to their colloidal dispersibility in dilute saline systems. Their large molecular dimensions render them easily retained within the sinus spaces and vascular elements, and thus not leaking away through bounding membranes. Other functions of hemocyanins, which in many instances may constitute the chief, if not indeed nearly the sole blood protein, include a principal role in maintaining a balanced colloidal osmotic pressure, perhaps thus precluding water losses otherwise risked due to blood hydrostatic pressures. As the chief blood protein, hemocyanin acts in the role of an amphoteric buffer, maintaining neutrality or normal pH levels against any environmentally induced variations in the pH of the body fluids. The same copper protein is able also to transport waste carbon dioxide for ultimate discharge, in a manner similar to its oxygen carriage, and to maintain the equilibrium of electrolytic systems separated by membranes, both those within the body and others in contact with marine, fresh, or brackish environmental waters.

Michael Pilson made some arresting observations anent the

wide ranges of hemocyanin concentrations in the plasma of
Haliotis abalone species. Whereas the lesser, nonhemocyanin
plasma protein from several *Haliotis* species exhibited but
minor variations in concentration, there were very wide differences in the hemocyanin levels, as follows.

	H. fulgens	*H. cracherodii*	*H. corrugata*
Non-HCy Protein			
Mean value %	0.20	0.14	0.24
HCy Protein %			
Low	0.03	0.21	0.0017
High	1.89	2.03	1.53
Median	0.54	0.38	0.15
Range	63-fold	10-fold	900-fold

A fourth species, *H. rufescens,* the red abalone, exhibited
similar wide variations in individual plasma hemocyanin concentrations.

Earlier studies on the blue crab *Callinectes sapidus,* by Hor-
ner and Kerr, had shown similar wide variations in plasma protein, both copper-combined and the other, nonmetallic type. A
10-fold variation in total serum protein concentration and an
18-fold range in quantities of bound copper were found. There
was no apparent correlation between size of crab and serum
protein or Cu concentrations, but a sexual difference was manifest in that females carried significantly more serum protein and
higher Cu concentrations than males. Females designated by the
investigators as being "in sponge" (egg-carrying), moreover,
had hemolymph considerably richer in hemocyanin than that of
unripe females.

Pilson's findings with the four abalone species indicated that
HCy concentrations were not correlated to weight, sex, reproductive season (by gonad index), nutritional condition, water
depth or habitat (collection site), or season of year.

While there can be no contradiction regarding the role of
hemocyanin as a reversible oxygen carrier, we must for the present agree with Pilson that the enormous ranges in hemocyanin
concentration in *Haliotis* plasma appear to lack compatibility

with any (other) physiological role thus far suggested. It remains a puzzle as to why individuals within a common marine animal species should vary in their respiratory oxygen-carrying copper protein by 10-, 60-, or even 900-fold.

These observations by Pilson on four abalone species, and by Horne and Kerr on the blue crab pose questions as to whether the animals indeed have an acute need for hemocyanin in substantial concentrations for meeting any of the several physiological requirements that it is reputed to serve. May it indeed be merely that the animals, assimilating considerable dissolved copper from their environment, link it to protein as a detoxicating device, and then utilize a part of the resulting complex to serve useful ends?

HEMERYTHRINS

These iron-bonding, colored protein types occur in the blood or blood cells of but a few invertebrate forms, including notably gephyrean worms of the genera *Sipunculus, Phascolosoma, Phymosoma* (or *Physcosoma*), and *Dendrostoma,* the polychaete annelid worm *Megalona,* and certain lingulid brachiopods such as *Lingula unguis.* The hemerythrin chromoproteins are of lower molecular weight than hemocyanins, and have been found to indicate values around 10.7×10^4, involving 16 Fe atoms per molecule, thus amounting to about 0.83 percent of the chromoprotein molecule. Oxyhemerythrin is brick-red to madder-red in color, showing spectral maxima at 280, 330, and 500 nm, the latter being the chief peak. In the reduced state, the compound is colorless to pale yellow, and shows no visible absorption bands.

Unlike the condition in hemoglobin, and recalling the case applying to hemocyanin, no porphyrin moiety exists as a binding link between the metallic ion and the protein in hemerythrin. There are reasons for supposing that each Fe atom is bonded to protein primarily through an imidazole N atom, and/or through a tyrosine residue. Like the hemoglobins and hemocyanins, hemerythrins involve globular proteins, peculiar to each species of animal carrying the pigment.

Hemerythrin purified by dialysis is barely acidic, manifesting pH levels between 5.8 and 6.0 and an isoelectric range between pH 4.8 and 5.7.

Hemerythrin analyses have indicated, for its chemical composition, the following proportions: C: 46.7%, H: 6.9%, N: 17.2%, S: 0.58%, Fe: from 0.51 to 1.44%, and presumably some 27 to 28% O by difference. It combines less readily with atmospheric oxygen than does hemoglobin, and requires less oxygen to saturate it. In contrast with hemoglobin and hemocyanin, it does not unite with either carbon monoxide or cyanide. A portion of the iron seems to be bonded rather loosely, becoming dissociated to yield the free ionized form merely on warming to mammalian blood temperatures, for example, 35-40°C. Any claim that hemerythrin is degraded by treatment with hydrogen sulfide presents an enigma when it is remembered that some of the sipunculid worms (e.g., *Dendrostoma zostericola*), equipped with the pigment, inhabit or assuredly visit anaerobic environments within sand or mud where this toxic chemical is manifestly present.

Not actually related to this respiratory pigment is an iron-transporting agent, ferritin, in which the iron is rather loosely bonded to a protein called transferrin or siderophilin, of molecular weight around 5×10^5, and thus retainable by the kidney. Ferritin is encountered in the mammalian gut wall, whence it is transferred along to the liver for further distribution. Ferritin permits loosely bonded ferric Fe^{3+} iron to be reduced enzymatically to soluble ferrous Fe^{2+} iron, and to be thus passed through the cell membrane into the blood, where, again restored to the Fe^{3+} state, it is rebonded to plasma globulin as transferrin.

HEMOVANADINS

It is under this heading that we encounter the most singular and enigmatic example of a metalloprotein, or indeed of any blood pigment. Should the "hemo" prefix perchance be taken to connote a known functional role within the blood, this would be misleading, since none is known at present; hence the prefix refers only to the common *site* of the biochrome. While minor levels of vanadium ions occur in the body fluids and tissues of certain molluscs and other marine invertebrates, it is among the ascidians or tunicates, of primitive chordate ilk, where we encounter the extraordinary vanadium chromoproteins. These are most commonly contained within minute, morula-shaped cells, the vanadocytes, each some 8 microns (μ) in diameter, or about that of an erythrocyte disc, and varying but little from species to species. The hemovanadin within these cells takes the form of some eight to ten relatively large, apple-green, rounded bodies constituting the metallic chromoprotein.

The uniqueness of vanadium's incorporation as a protein-bonded ion is accompanied by yet another, equally extraordinary feature—that of the inclusion within the vanadocytes of free sulfuric acid, in concentrations, withal, as high as 9 percent, or nearly 2 normal. Neither the physiological significance of the vanadium complex nor that of the sulfuric acid has yet been established.

The green chromogen exhibits strongly reducing properties; it turns first brown, and ultimately dark blue-green, following cytolysis and resulting exposure to atmospheric oxygen. Also, on treatment with another strong oxidizing agent, osmium tetroxide, the chromogen instantly manifests a deep, blue-black appearance, not assignable to presence of lipids. The dark blue-green precipitate generated by atmospheric oxidation of the cytolyzed hemovanadin, and referred to as vanadochrome, has shown approximately the following chemical composition: C: 38.96%, H: 4.63%, N: 7.45%, and V: 10.08%, supposedly leaving some 38.88% O. Other analyses have indicated lower values for vanadium, about 5.51% and somewhat elevated figures for nitrogen, for example, 10.10%.

The initial brown chromogen vanadochrome, having undergone some oxidation, still is reducing in behavior, and is able, for example, to catalyze the oxidation of certain organic compounds, such as aniline and hydroquinone. The chromogen, separated from its protein conjugant, indicated no presence of purines, proteins, or amino acids, but was found to possess a considerable pyrrole content; moreover, although indicating a molecular weight of about 900, the compound was diffusible through a collodion membrane. No porphyrin or cyclic tetra-pyrrole structure has been detected, but there may be chains of linear tetrapyrroles (bilichromes) involved. Indeed, the observed primary appearance of the red-brown colored chromogen, followed by its oxidation to a blue-green phase, are suggestive of the possible sequential manifestations of bilirubin and its oxidized product biliverdin, both perhaps still conjugated or chelated in some way with vanadium and organic radicals.

From what is currently known, it appears that the vanadium is in the reduced, so-called vanadyl V^{2+} state as bonded, through its chromogen partner, to protein within the vanadocytes; that, upon cytolysis and resulting exposure of the contents to air, the V ion progresses to the next (reddish-brown) stage of oxidation, V^{3+}, and finally, at the dark-blue or blue-green stage, to the V^{4+} valence, not present in the intact cells. Presumably the high intracellular acidity stabilizes the reduced V^{2+} condition while linked to the protein within the vanadocytes. Under these same intracellular acidic conditions, the hemovanadin is able to reduce cellular cytochrome c; it is capable also of reducing added methylene blue, both aerobically and anaerobically.

No physiological function has been recognized for hemovanadin. The earlier view that it might serve as a respiratory aid or catalyst has been abandoned. High oxygen tensions induce the dissolution of no more of the gas in tunicate blood containing vanadocytes than in the same volume of seawater. Nor is the hemovanadin capable of serving as a reversible hydrogen acceptor. Moreover, seawater solutions of ferrous salts, sulfite, thiosulfate, iodide, or glucose are oxidized by atmospheric oxygen bubbles no more readily in the presence of vanadocytes than in control systems without them.

Ascidians, equipped with their extensive respiratory surfaces, hardly would appear to require a special oxygen transporter or other respiratory biochrome.

Furthermore, certainly not all tunicate species possess hemovanadin. The absence of respiratory biochromes (save for the universal cytochromes), characterizes many other invertebrates, including coelenterates, echinoderms, most bivalves and opisthobranch molluscs, and even a far more metabolically active group, the insects, which inhabit regions of higher and more changeable temperatures.

We are confronted by the riddle of how evolutionary processes have endowed some tunicate species with the capacity to assimilate and bind vanadium, as well as sulfuric acid, while allowing other species within the same subphylum to develop without this synthetic capacity, or perhaps to lose it.

Seawater, bearing some 0.3 to 0.6 mg of vanadium per cubic meter, must be the chief source supplying the metallic ion to the ceaselessly filtering ascidians. A large (15-cm long) specimen of *Ascidia,* placed in seawater fortified with vanadium ion to a level of 0.65 mg per l (or approximately 1,000-fold its natural quantity) has been observed to remove about 4.2 μg V per hour. Vanadium salts in seawater readily become adsorbed to, or incorporated in, the mucous sheet covering the exposed branchial apparatus and in the gut, for example, of both *Ascidia ceratodes,* which possesses vanadocytes, and *Ciona intestinalis,* which does not. Both species transport vanadium via the ovary into the developing ova. Two species of *Styela* yield no V, while *Euherdmania clavicornis* has been found to store 475, and *Ciona intestinalis* 100 p.p.m. There is firm ground for the view that soluble or colloidally dispersed vanadium compounds constitute a common and available source of the metal for these sea squirts. There always remains the possibility that enriched V concentrations may occur in various small planktonic organisms or in finely particulate detritus, representing the kind of materials continually taken into the alimentary tract of ascidians.

ADENOCHROME

When for the first time one cuts open the visceral dome, a large, saclike body above the mouth and eye head parts of an octopus, for example, *O. bimaculatus,* one encounters yet another chromatic surprise, quite apart from the rapid blueing of the shed blood. That is, one sees a pair of small, ovoid purple pulsating hearts lying externally of the large kidney sac, one at the base of each gill. These two organs are equipped with muscles, serving to pump blood into the gills, but are, moreover, constituted largely of spongy, glandular tissue, and likely exercise an excretory function for fluid wastes.

In a cephalopod mollusc, which carries in its circulatory fluid no hemoglobin or other visible iron-bearing protein—indeed no visibly colored substance at all, but only colorless (reduced) cuprous hemocyanin—why or how do these branchial hearts manifest a purple color, strongly suggestive of an iron-bearing entity? Admittedly, our first view of the pigmented tissue in an animal lacking hemoglobin exercised another turn of the screw.

David Updegraff and I found the answer to be that an iron complex is in fact involved, but in a stable, sparingly soluble, bonded ferric condition. Microscopic inspection of the tissue reveals myriads of garnet-red, microspheroid inclusions, stored within the glandular cells, and believed to constitute a metabolic waste product.

When cut, the tissue yields its now exposed pigment slowly to water, but quite readily to dilute ammonia or other alkalis. Such aqueous extracts afford deep-wine-red colloidal solutions, exhibiting the Tyndall cone of scattered light when illuminated by a narrow beam. The pigment in such solutions does not diffuse through membranes, for example, into distilled water, and is not precipitated either by boiling temperatures or by saturation of the system with sodium chloride, or even with ammonium sulfate, the usual precipitating agent for protein systems. Acidification, even mildly, to a pH value of 5.75, or the addition of small amounts of alcohol or acetone, effects a color change from the wine-red to a cloudy purple, with final precipitation of all the pigment as amorphous purple flocs.

This extraordinary pigment (which we were the first to describe, and which we named adenochrome for its presence in glandular tissue) may amount to from 11 to 37 percent of the branchial heart tissue, on a dry-weight basis. It is recoverable by repeated precipitation with alcohol, yielding a noncrystalline, mauve or purplish powder that withstands temperatures up to 300°C without melting or showing visible decomposition, but which chars at higher temperatures. It is insoluble not only in alcohol but in ether, chloroform, dioxane, or glacial acetic acid, dissolving somewhat in pure trichloracetic acid and in dilute pyridine, the latter thus behaving as a weakly alkaline fluid, like dilute ammonia.

Adenochrome in dilute alkaline solution exhibits a single,

broad spectral absorption maximum, centering close to 505 nm. It is bleached to a pale yellow color on mixing with hyposulfite, but is readily reoxidized to the red condition by aeration. The red compound is adsorbable from aqueous systems by magnesium or calcium oxides, but not by talc, kaolin, starch, or alumina. Not unexpectedly, the pigment is irreversibly oxidized by powerful reagents such as concentrated nitric or sulfuric acids, permanganate, or bromine. It also is readily reduced by zinc dust in alkali, which affords a ready source of nascent hydrogen.

Roasting of the purified and dried material emits the familiar odor of burning feathers (characteristic of proteins) and gives a positive reaction for pyrroles by reddening a pine splinter moistened with concentrated HCl, then exposed to the fumes.

Aqueous solutions of adenochrome respond strongly to the ninhydrin test for a-amino groups or alkyl amines. Its further simulation of protein is manifest in its precipitability by dialyzed colloidal iron oxide, salts of heavy metals such as copper, lead, mercury, or silver, and from neutral solution by the so-called alkaloidal reagents, including dilute phosphotungstic, phosphomolybdic, or picric acids. It responds by but a feebly positive reaction, however, to the biuret test for indicating —CONH— linkages.

In other respects adenochrome exhibits marked contrasts to protein, for example, in affording no coagulum or precipitate in boiling water, and in giving precipitates with alcohol or acetone, as do proteins, but, unlike them, readily redissolving in cold, dilute alkali. It also responds *negatively* to certain standard tests for protein, such as the xanthoproteic reaction with concentrated nitric acid (with which protein gives a bright yellow color), followed by alkalization with ammonia (whereupon the color changes to orange-red), for phenolic groups; Millon's or Sakaguchi's reaction; the aldehyde test for tryptophan; or the alkaline lead test for reduced sulfur. The above-mentioned solubility of adenochrome in trichloracetic acid also is completely nontypical of any protein; indeed proteins are precipitated by the reagent.

The yield of ash from total ignition of the purified, dry adenochrome has shown variations, ranging from about 4.2 to 7.4

percent, and the raw pigment contains from 0.43 to 0.67 percent iron, seemingly all in the fully oxidized Fe^{3+} state. Thus if 5.8 percent may represent the average ash content, and 0.55 percent the mean value for iron content, this would signify the iron content of ash to be just short of 10 percent. The roughly 0.55 percent of iron in adenochrome exceeds that of hemoglobin (about 0.33 percent), and is far short of that in ferritin (20-22 percent), the iron-storing protein in mammalian bone marrow which conserves the iron from hemoglobin breakdown, and hence for recycling in newly generated hemoglobin.

The elementary composition of ash-free adenochrome corresponds to the following approximate proportions: C: 41.33%, H: 5.98%, N: 13.8%, S: 5.67%, and O (by difference): 33.72%. The nearest tentative empirical formula was thus worked out as follows: $C_{41}H_{72}N_{12}O_{25}S_2$, with a minimum molecular weight close to 1200.

Adenochrome apparently carries nearly 3% N in a-amino and/or alkyl amine status, between approximately 4 and 7% as amide-N, and comparable amounts as imidazole-bonded N.

Thus in its elementary chemical makeup, adenochrome has been compared with the yellow, excretory melanoid substance, urochrome, conspicuous in and recoverable from mammalian urine. It resembles urochrome also in its insolubility in alcohol and other fat solvents, its solubility in trichloracetic acid, its yielding of pyrrolic materials during destructive roasting, and its precipitability by heavy metal salts and by the alkaloidal reagents named.

But there are certain striking contrasts as well. For example, whereas both of these excretory substances appear to carry nearly the same proportions of combined sulfur, all of this element is firmly bound and in the oxidized state in adenochrome, whereas in urochrome reduced sulfur can be released readily on exposure to warm alkali, and demonstrated by adding lead ion to give the black sulfide.

Again, while eight hours "hydrolysis" of urochrome with 6N HCl yielded quantitative amounts of uromelanin, hydrolysis of adenochrome for eight hours with 33% sulfuric acid afforded but a little brown sediment, leaving the principal chemical properties unchanged.

Finally, exposure of adenochrome to strong, concentrated alkali evokes the evolution of ammonia (and/or similar volatile amines), suggesting the possibility that the alkaline, nitrogenous radicals might be linked with acidic sulfonate groups to give the corresponding salts.

We regard adenochrome as a catabolic, nitrogenous waste product, notably in view of the presence of much labile ammonium or amide nitrogen stored by the molecule in a readily alkaline-hydrolyzable status. The material may thus serve as a kind of reservoir, keeping free catabolic ammonia and kindred amines beneath the toxic level in the animal's body. The presence of imidazole likewise may indicate that adenochrome serves as an excretory material similar or analogous to urochrome, the yellow waste substance in mammalian urine. The presence of fully oxidized sulfur in adenochrome suggests not only its likely identity as a catabolic end product but also the possibility of an operative detoxicating function similar to those reactions which occur in mammalian systems, wherein certain poisonous molecules are convertible into innocuous sulfonates or other derivatives involving oxidized forms of sulfur. Examples of this are to be found, inter alia, in the detoxication of phenolic substances or toxic products of intestinal putrefaction, by their metabolic conversion into sulfates or sulfonates, in which form they are excreted in mammalian urine as so-called ethereal sulfates; another instance is the presence of thiocyanate (CNS^-) ion in adult human saliva, which presumably represents the body's method of detoxicating traces of cyanide, fortuitously assimilated in the consumption of certain fruits or of breathing contaminated fumes, such as tobacco smoke.

We remained puzzled to have encountered adenochrome solely in the glandular tissues of the paired gill hearts of the cephalopod and not in the adjacent excretory nephridial gland that invested the vena cava, supplying blood to the gills through the hearts. However, no efficient means of eliminating the pigmentary substance itself seemed feasible, since adenochrome indeed is a slightly acidic substance, soluble only in alkaline media, and not at all in even mildly acidic systems. The pH level of freshly cut and exposed gill-heart tissue shows an average value of about 5.0, a feature affording an unfavorable condition for dissolution of the compound, or resultant transportation in its precipitated form within the cells.

It may be that the accumulation of catabolic adenochrome within the cells of the branchial hearts constitutes a natural limitation upon the life-span of the octopus.

We later encountered in the ruddy-colored bryozoan *Bugula neritina* a biochrome resembling adenochrome in some features, but certainly distinct from it. This pigment, first described by the previously mentioned Gilberto Villela, occurs as ellipsoid or irregularly shaped, microscopic granular plastids within the distal parts of the zooecium, and around the so-called brown body, believed to be associated with waste storage and/ or disposal. We recovered 21 mg of the pigment from a 36-g colony of *Bugula* (wet weight), by extracting in boiling water. The extract proved wine-red in color and gave a pH value of about 6.8. In contrast to adenochrome, the *Bugula* pigment was precipitated by potassium hydroxide, and redissolved in 10% acetic acid. Moreover, it displayed a sharp absorption peak at 545 nm, instead of adenochrome's broad, rounded maximum centering at 505 nm.

Like adenochrome, the *Bugula* pigment was observed to be sorbable by oxides of magnesium or calcium, although it also was firmly adherent to alumina; moreover, it was oxidized by permanganate or hydrogen peroxide, reducible by hyposulfite or by alkalized zinc dust, and was negative in response to the xanthoproteic and biuret tests. The murexide reaction for purines and the Salkowski test for indole also were negative, as with adenochrome, which, however, yielded pyrroles on roasting. The *Bugula* product reacted positively to the ninhydrin test, emitted ammonia or other volatile amines on treatment with concentrated alkali, and gave no evidence of the presence of reduced sulfur. These still puzzling, suspectedly excretory colored compounds call for more study. And this last-mentioned desideratum does not, as L-G remarks, add much if anything to set them far apart from the rest of the diversified biochrome family. Finally, she does agree that these enigmatic biochromes, like a bulging purse discovered in one's path, invite looking into.

Appendix

CAROTENOIDS

α-Carotene

$C_{40}H_{56}$

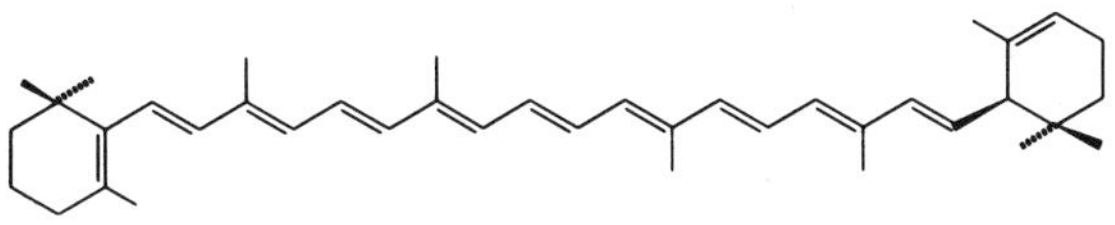

1

β-Carotene

$C_{40}H_{56}$

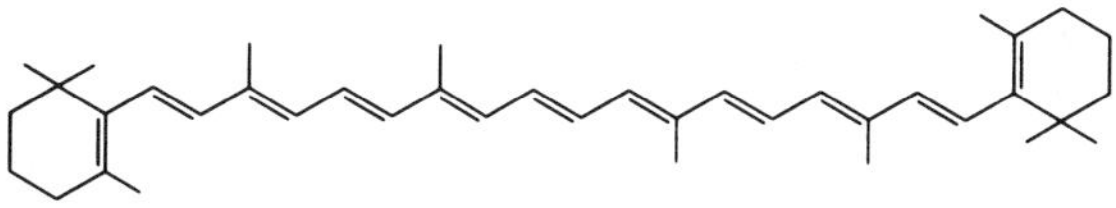

2

γ-Carotene

$C_{40}H_{56}$

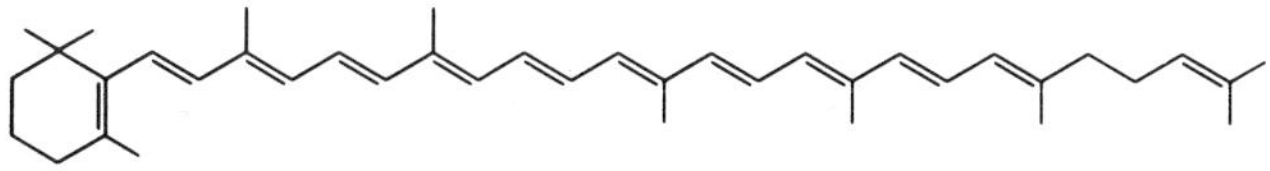

3

ε-Carotene

$C_{40}H_{56}$

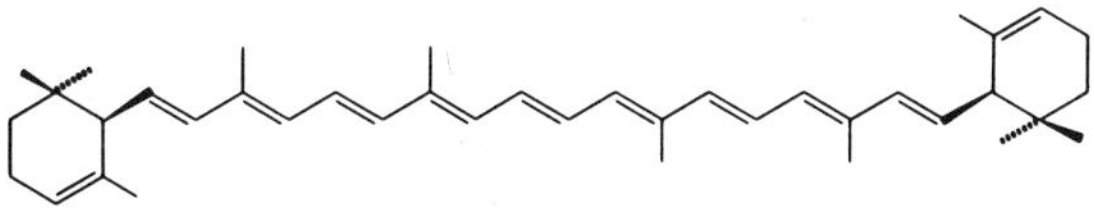

4

Lycopene

$C_{40}H_{56}$

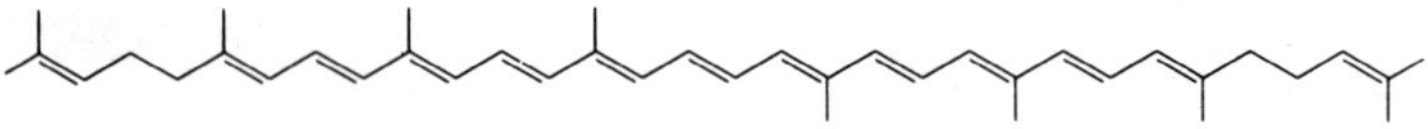

5

β-Cryptoxanthin.

$C_{40}H_{56}O$

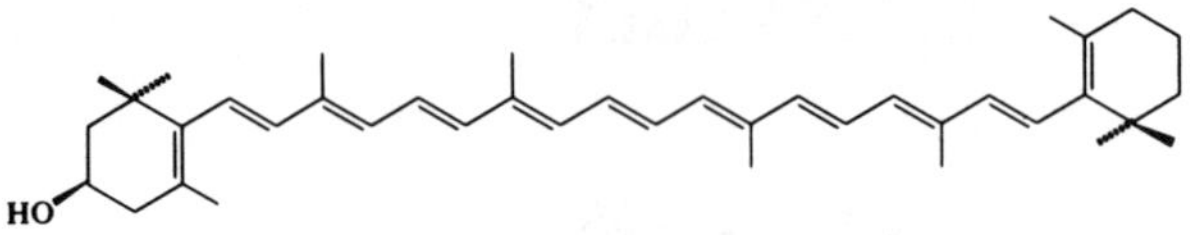

6

Lutein.

$C_{40}H_{56}O_2$

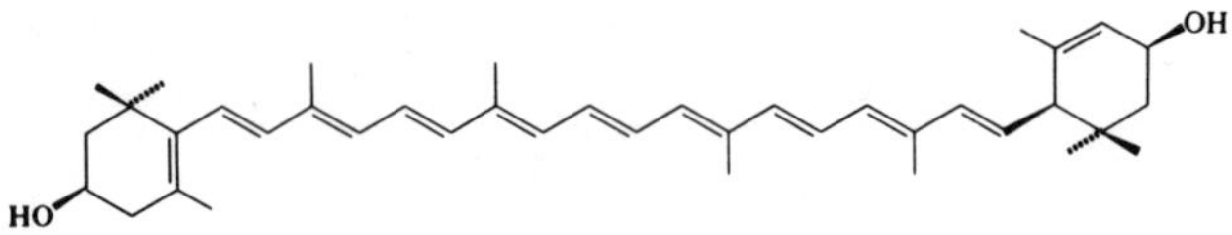

7

Zeaxanthin

$C_{40}H_{56}O_2$

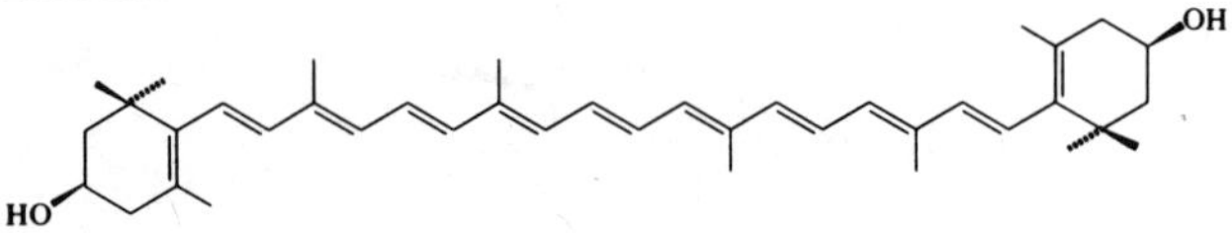

8

Isozeaxanthin

$C_{40}H_{56}O_2$

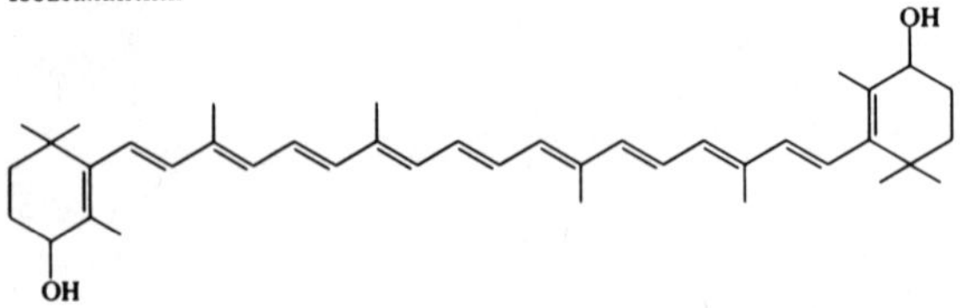

9

Tunaxanthin

$C_{40}H_{56}O_2$

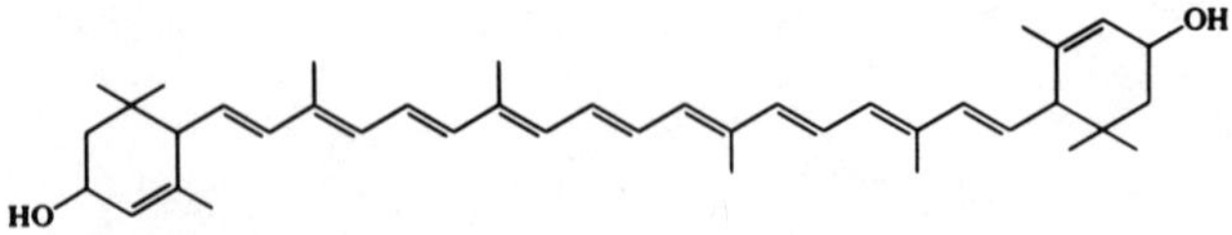

10

Taraxanthin

$C_{40}H_{56}O_3$

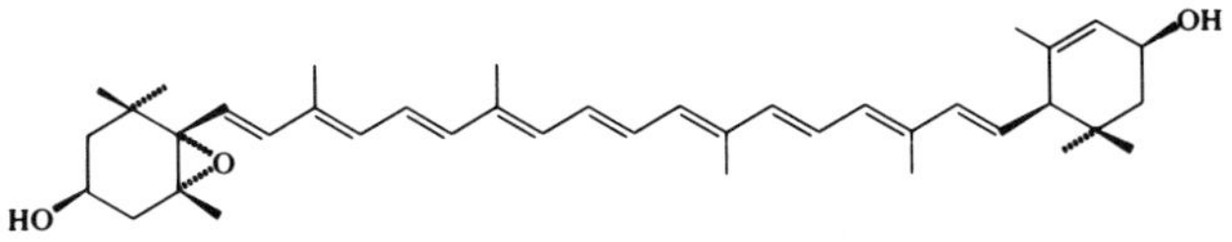

11

Violaxanthin

$C_{40}H_{56}O_4$

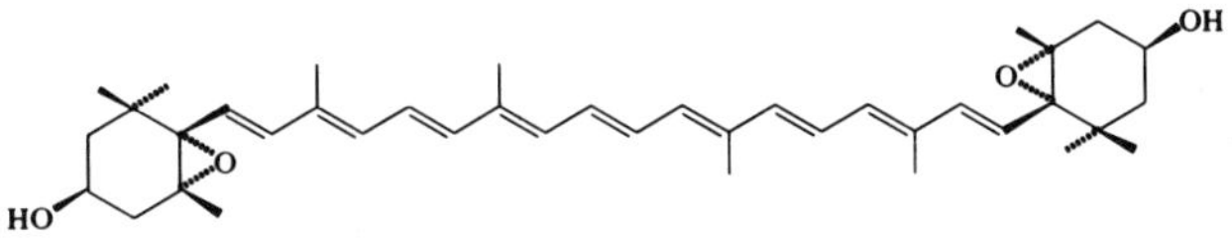

12

Fucoxanthinol

$C_{40}H_{56}O_5$

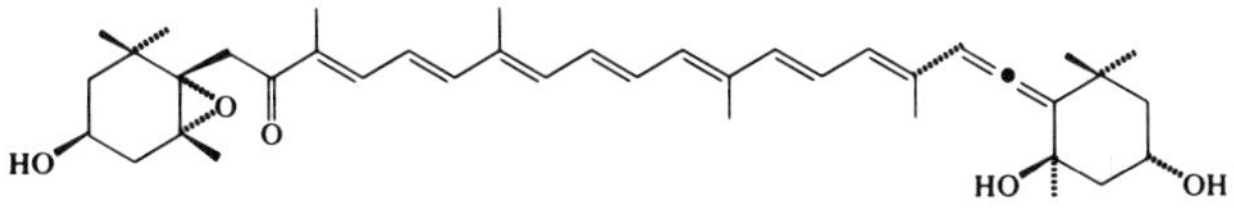

13

Fucoxanthin

$C_{42}H_{58}O_6$

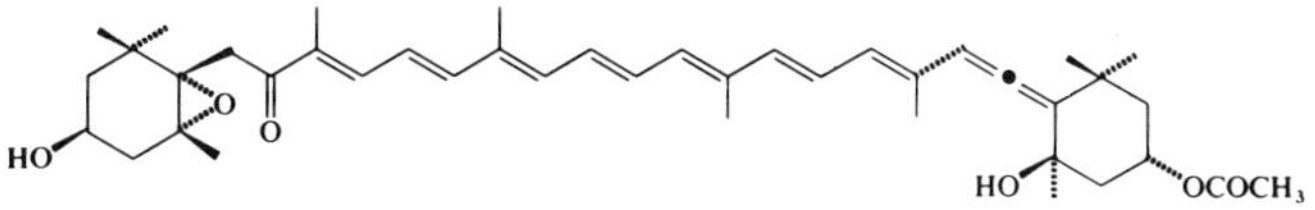

14

Diatoxanthin

$C_{40}H_{54}O_2$

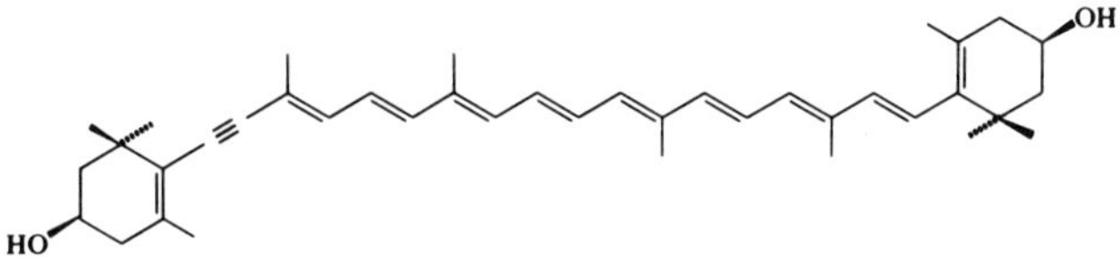

15

Diadinoxanthin

$C_{40}H_{54}O_3$

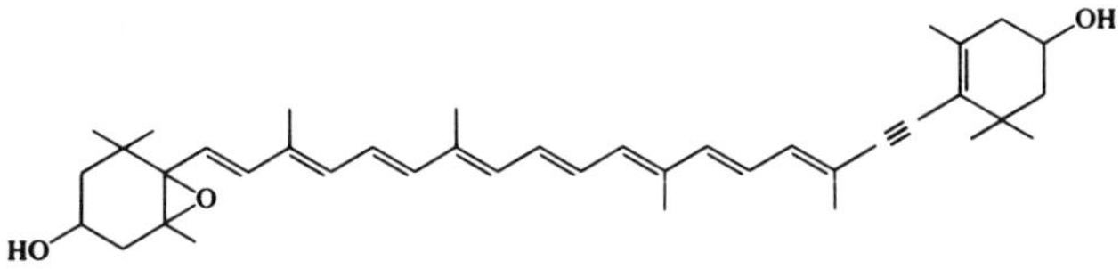

16

APPENDIX

Alloxanthin

$C_{40}H_{52}O_2$

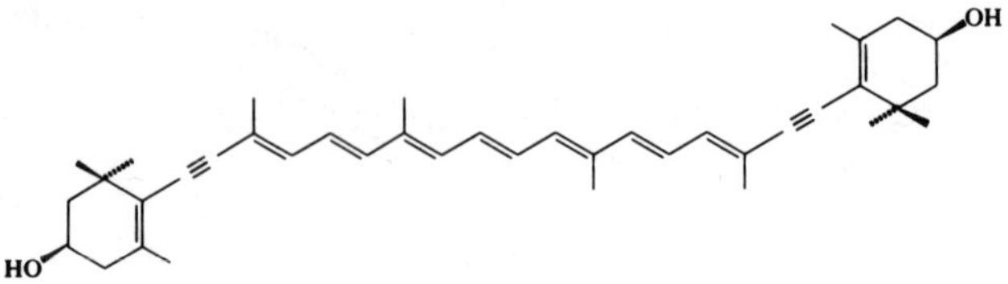

17

Peridinin,

$C_{39}H_{50}O_7$

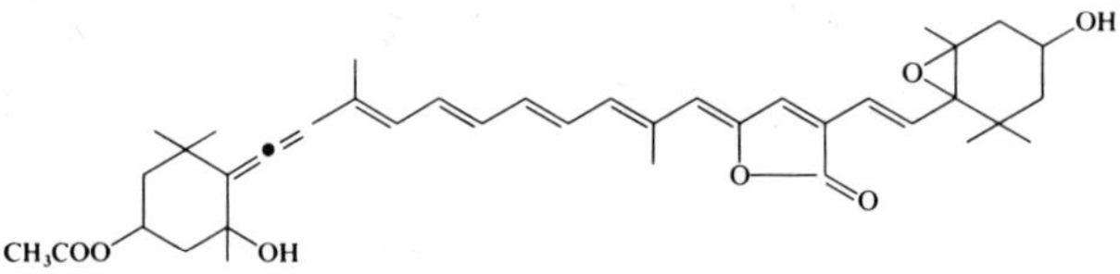

18

Echinenone

$C_{40}H_{54}O$

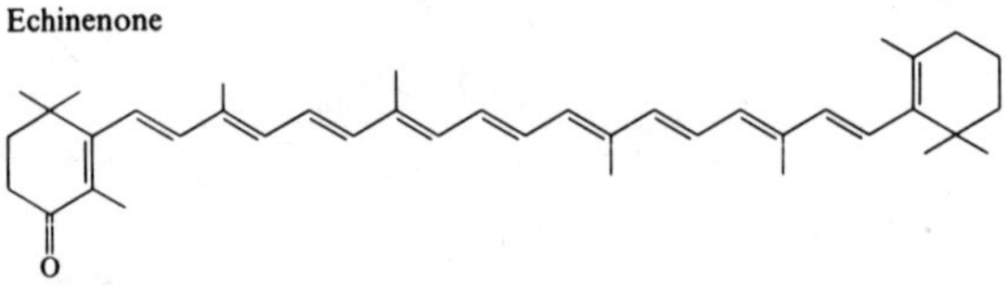

19a

Phoenicopterone

$C_{40}H_{54}O$

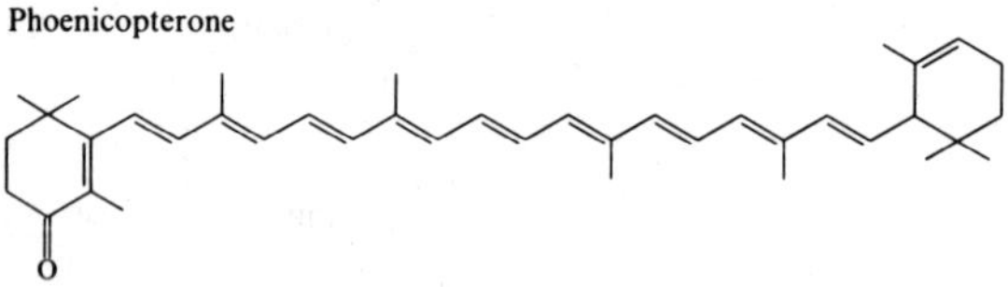

19b

Canthaxanthin

$C_{40}H_{52}O_2$

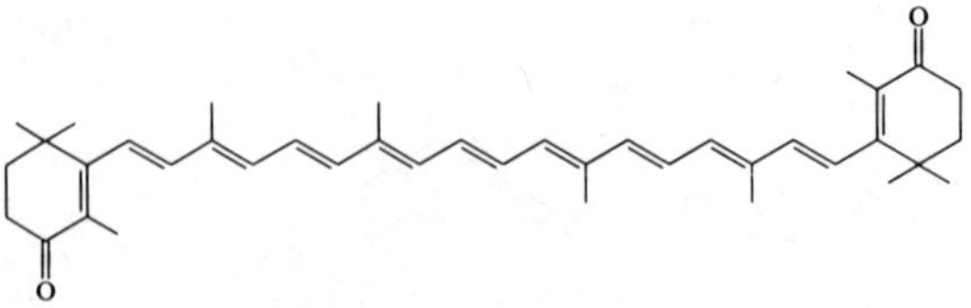

20

Phoenicoxanthin

$C_{40}H_{52}O_3$

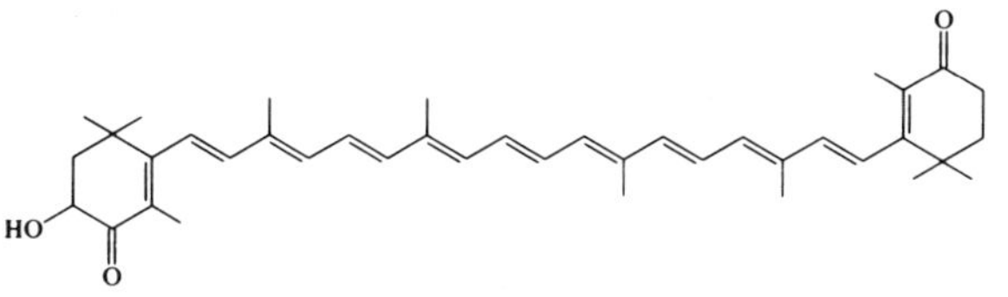

21

Astaxanthin,

$C_{40}H_{52}O_4$

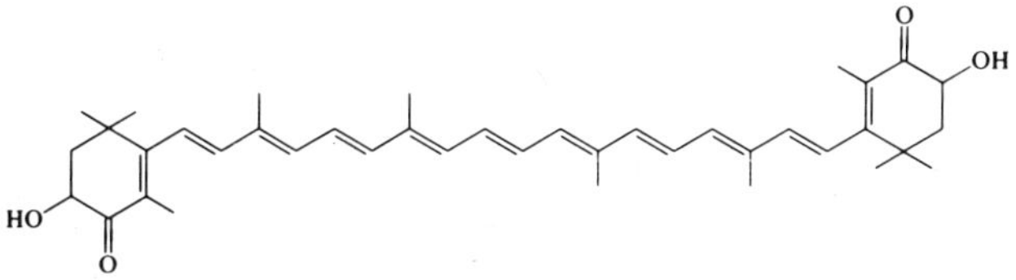

22

Astacene.

$C_{40}H_{48}O_4$

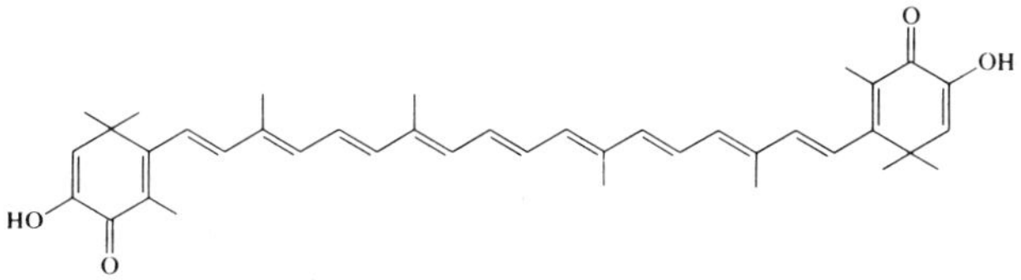

23

Actinioerythrin

$C_{38}H_{48}O_4$
(as diol)

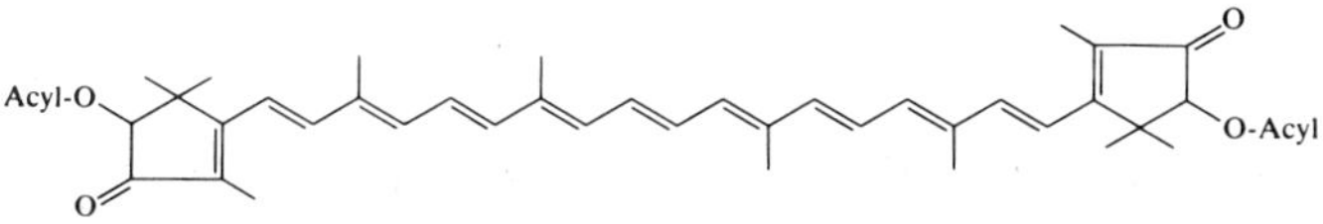

24

Capsanthin

$C_{40}H_{56}O_3$

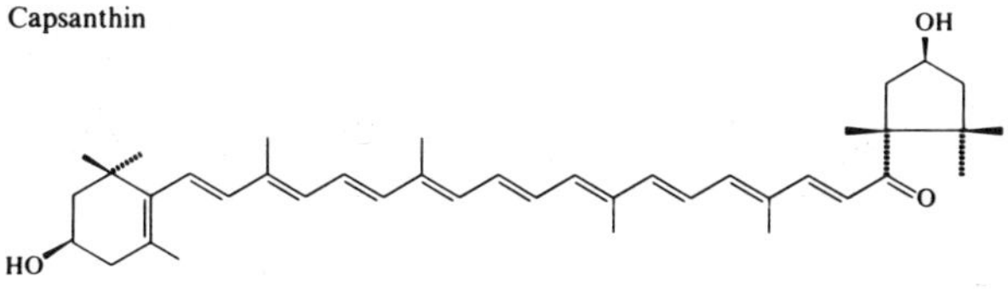

25

Hopkinsiaxanthin

$C_{31}H_{38}O_3$

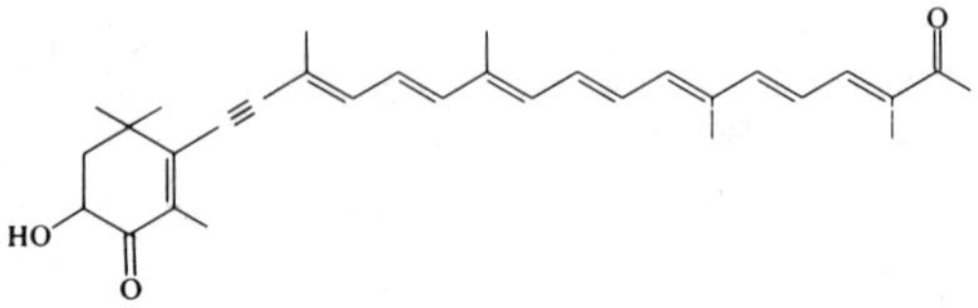

26

Renieratene

$C_{40}H_{48}$

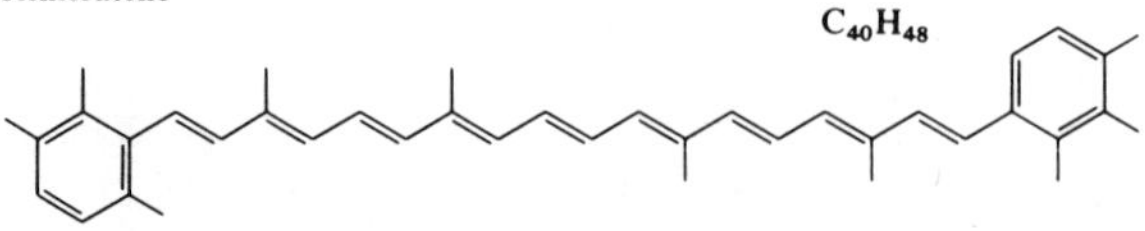

27

Isorenieratene

$C_{40}H_{48}$

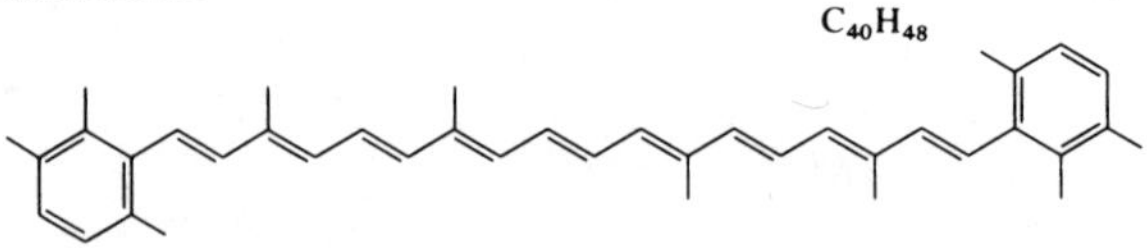

28

Renierapurpurin

$C_{40}H_{48}$

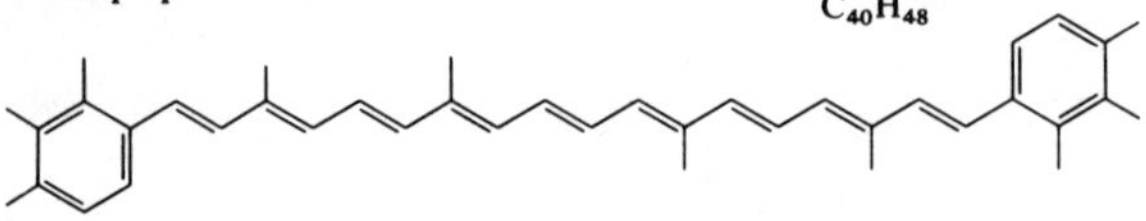

29

Aromatic
carotenoid
hydrocarbons

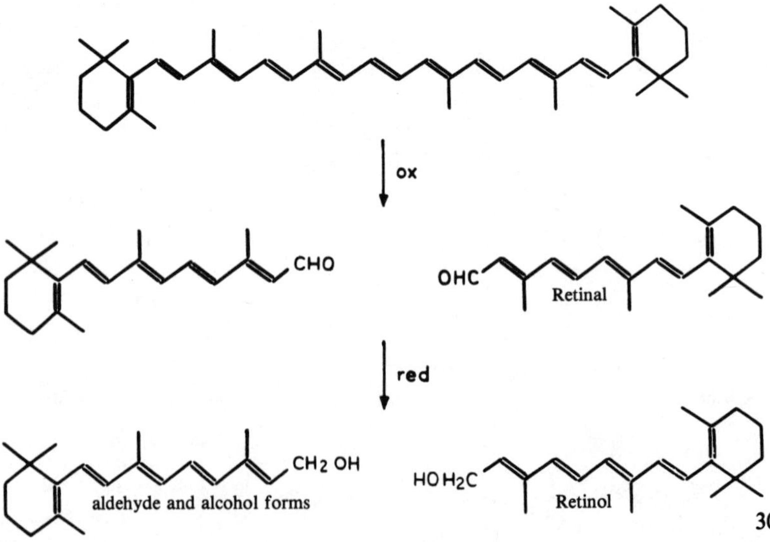

ox

CHO

OHC   Retinal

red

CH₂OH

aldehyde and alcohol forms

HOH₂C   Retinol

30

Enzymic genesis of A-vitamins from β-carotene

QUINONES

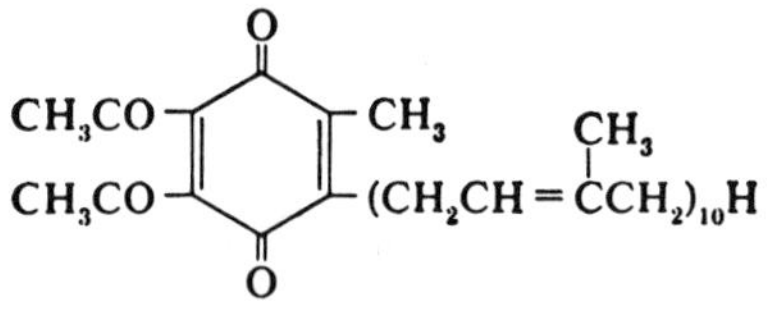

CH_3CO —⎡ O ⎤— CH_3 CH_3

CH_3CO —⎣ O ⎦— $(CH_2CH=CCH_2)_{10}H$

[ubiquinone (50)] or coenzyme Q_{10}

31

32

H H   OH O
HO—C—C ⎡   ⎤ OH
H H ⎣   ⎦
HO   OH
OH O

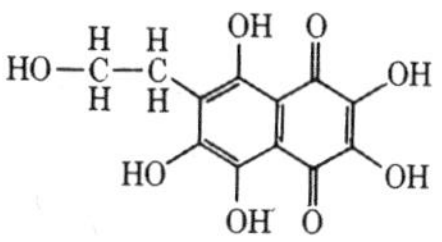

Echinochrome A
$C_{12}H_{10}O_8$

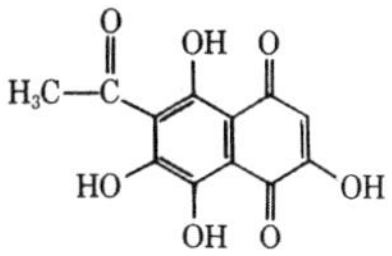

33

O   OH O
H_3C—C ⎡   ⎤
HO   OH
OH O

Spinochrome A
$C_{12}H_8O_7$

O   OH
⎡   ⎤ OH

O

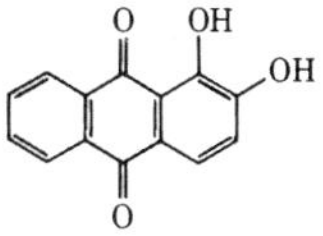

34

Alizarin (1, 2-dihydroxy-9,10-anthraquinone)

Vitamin K₁

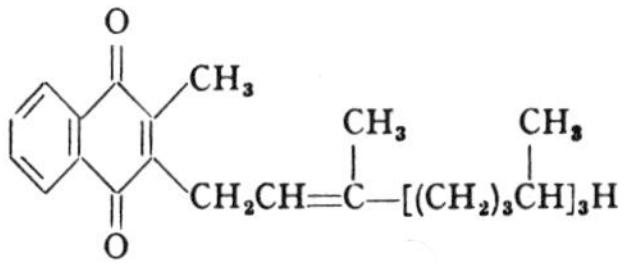

O
⎡   ⎤ CH_3 CH_3 CH_3
⎣   ⎦ $CH_2CH=C—[(CH_2)_3CH]_3H$
O

35

Vitamin K₂(₃₅)

O   n = 6
⎡   ⎤ CH_3 CH_3 CH_3
⎣   ⎦ $CH_2[CH=C(CH_2)_2]_nCH=C—CH_3$
O

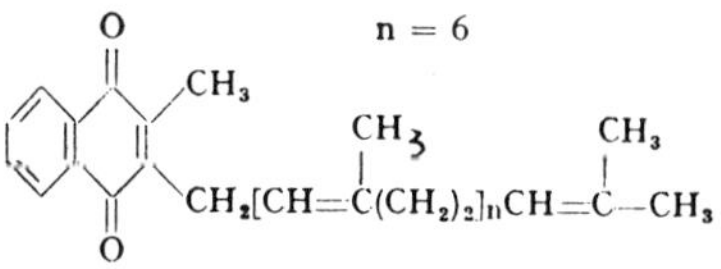

36

Rhodocomatulin-6-methyl-ether

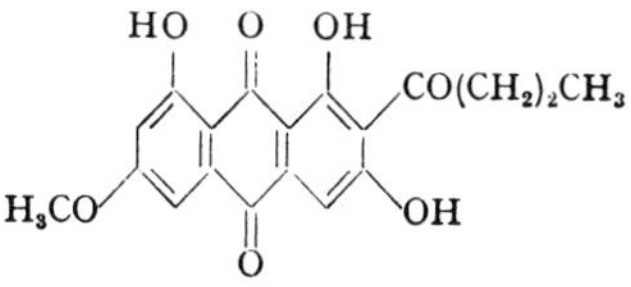

HO   O   OH
⎡   ⎤ $CO(CH_2)_4CH_3$
H_3CO OH
O

37

FLAVONOIDS

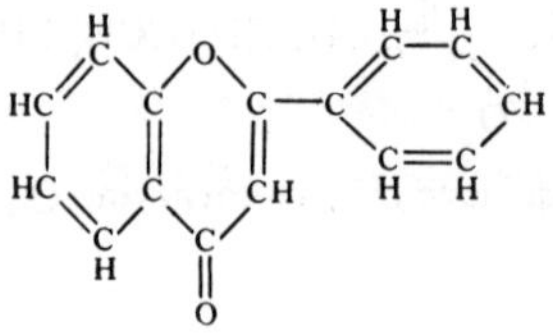

Flavone

38

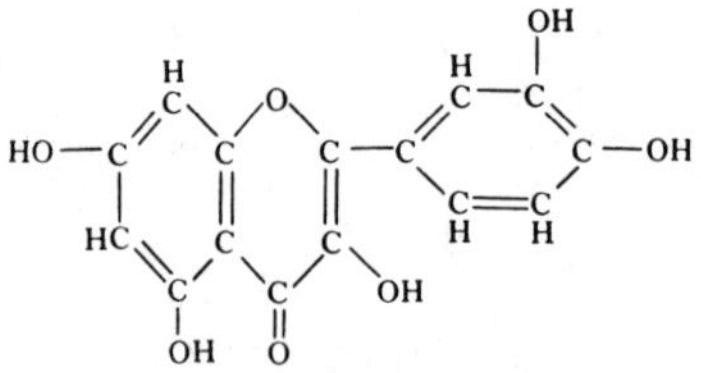

Quercitin

39

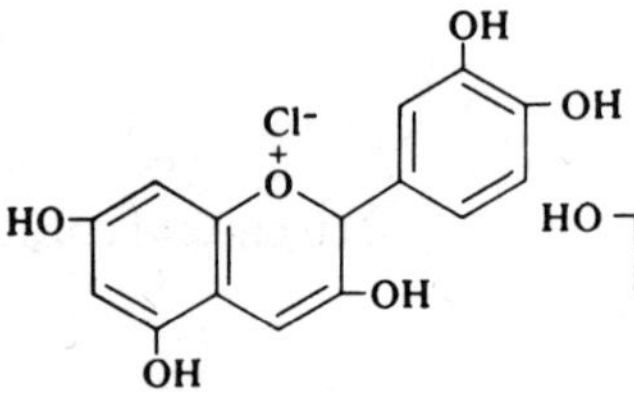

cyanidin chloride 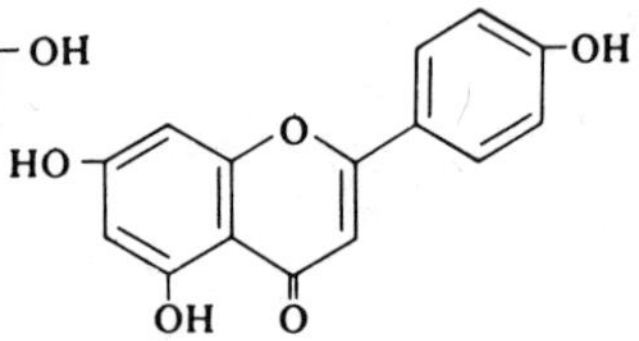   apigenin

40

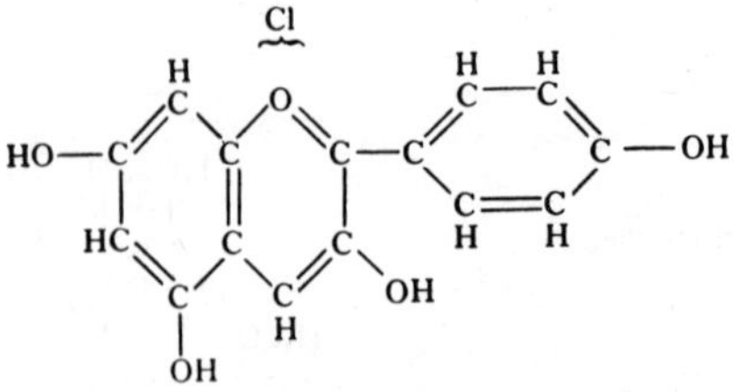

Pelargonidin chloride

41

QUINONES

Kermesic acid

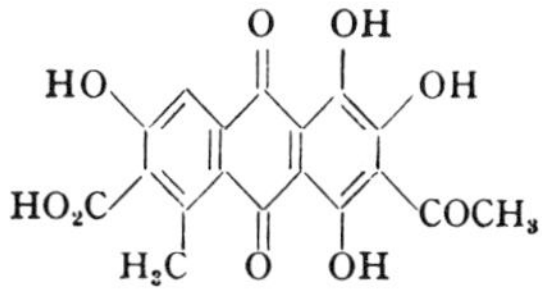

42

Carminic acid

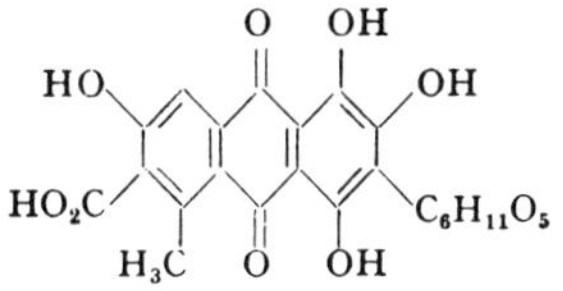

43

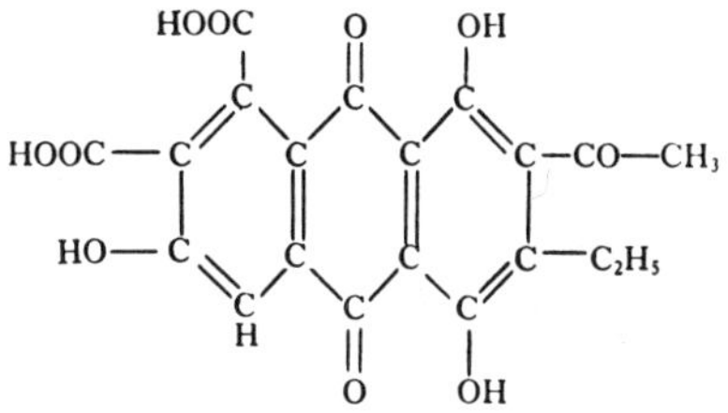

Laccaic acid

44

Protoaphin

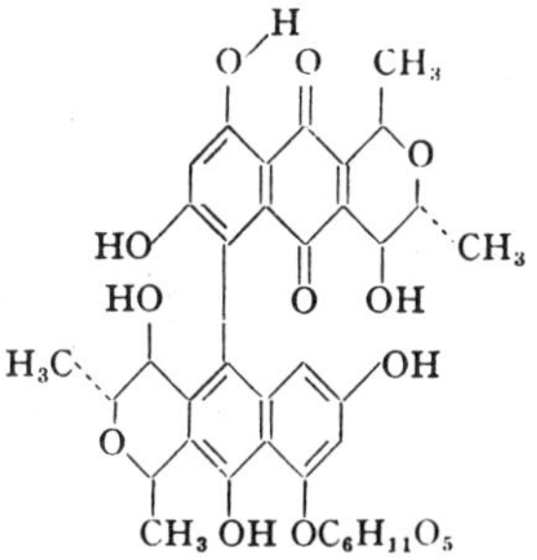

45

Erythroaphin

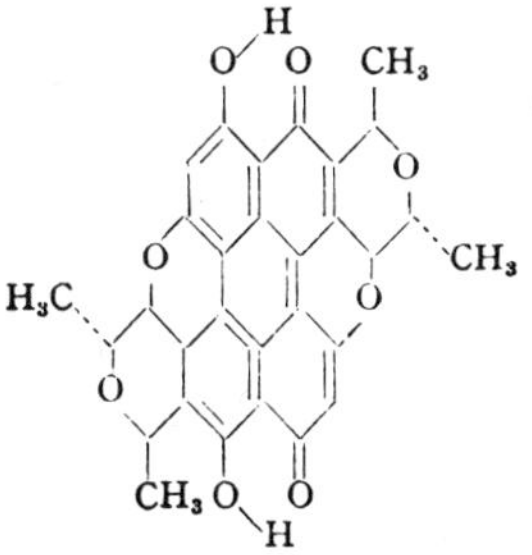

46

INDIGOIDS, MELANINS, and OMMOCHROMES

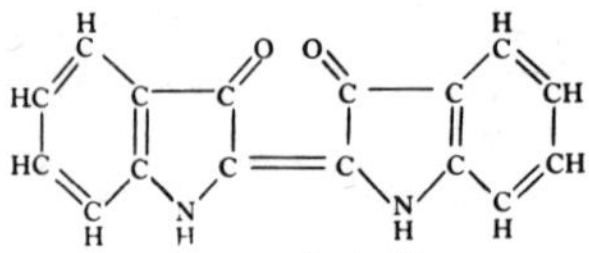

Indigotin

47

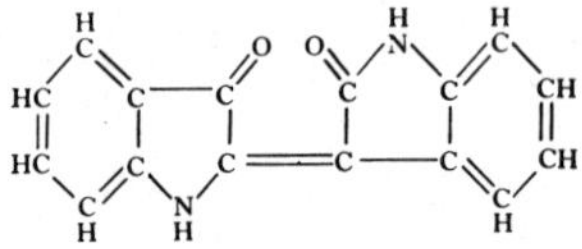

Indirubin

48

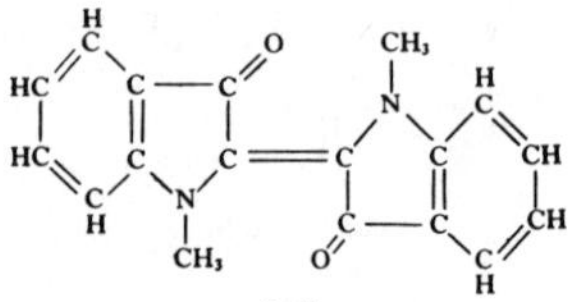

Indigo green

49

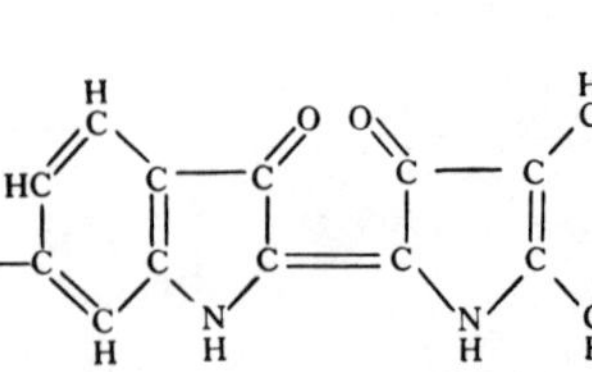

Leuco-indigo

50

Dibromindigo

51

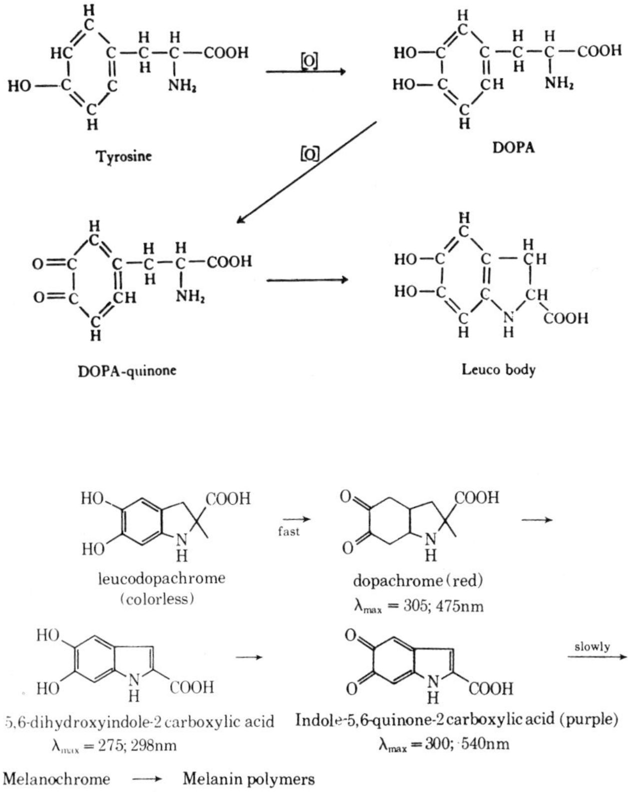

Tyrosine

[O]

[O]

DOPA

DOPA-quinone

Leuco body

leucodopachrome
(colorless)

fast

dopachrome (red)
$\lambda_{max} = 305; 475nm$

5,6-dihydroxyindole-2 carboxylic acid
$\lambda_{max} = 275; 298nm$

Indole-5,6-quinone-2 carboxylic acid (purple)
$\lambda_{max} = 300; 540nm$

slowly

Melanochrome   ⟶   Melanin polymers

52

Melanin Formation

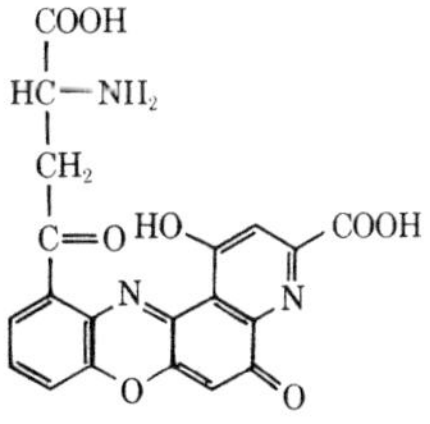

53

Xanthommatin

TETRAPYRROLES

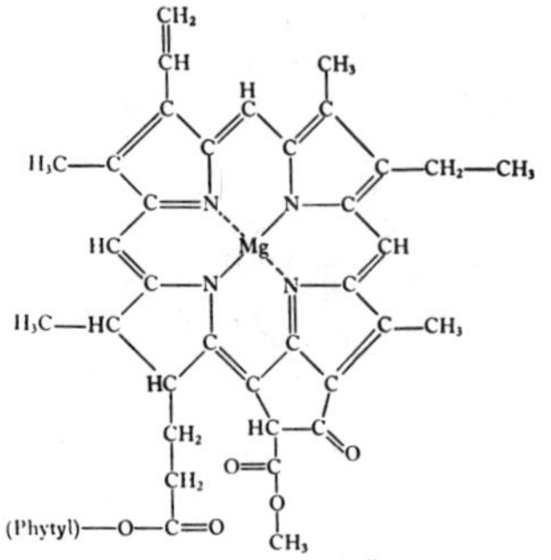

Chlorophyll-*a*

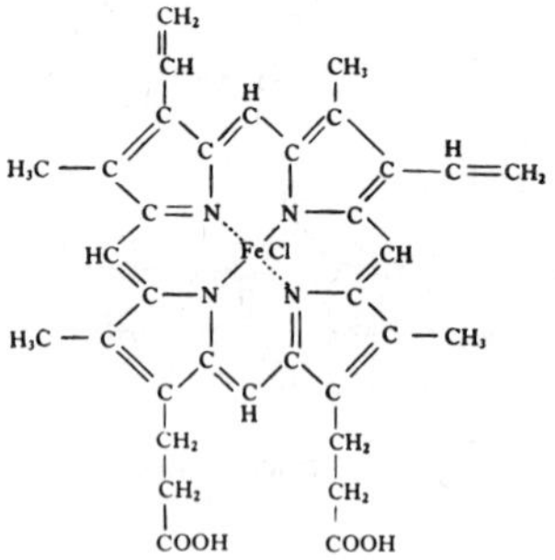

54

Hemin

55

PORPHYRINS

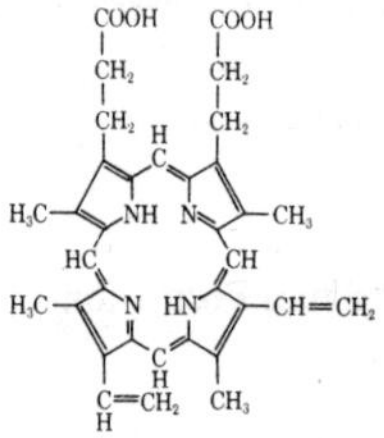

56

Protoporphyrin IX (= 1,3,5,8-Tetramethyl-2,4-divinylporphin-6,7-dipropionic acid)

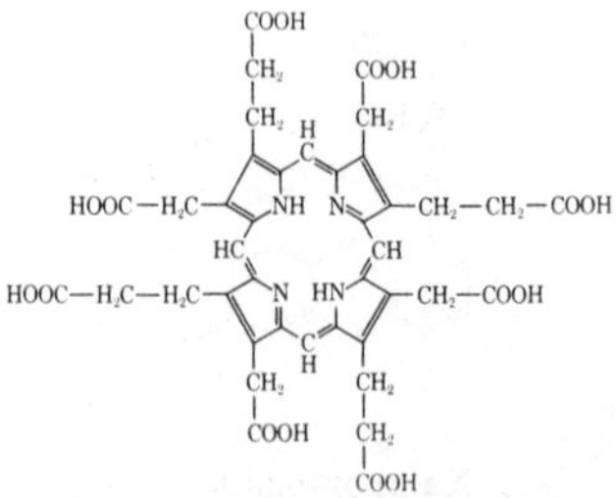

57

Uroporphyrin I (= Porphin-1,3,5,7-tetra-acetic-2,4,6,8-tetrapropionic acid)
(Uroporphyrin III is Porphin-1,3,5,8-tetra-acetic-2,4,6,7-tetrapropionic acid)

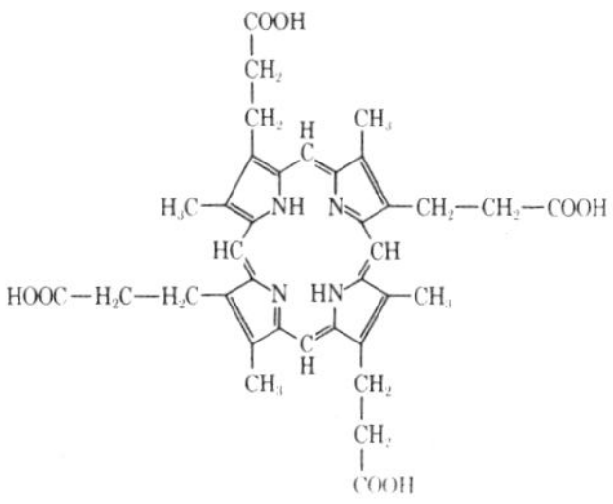

58

Coproporphyrin I (= 1,3,5,7-Tetramethylporphin-2,4,6,8-tetrapropionic acid)
(Coproporphyrin III is 1,3,5,8-Tetramethylporphin-2,4,6,7-tetrapropionic acid)

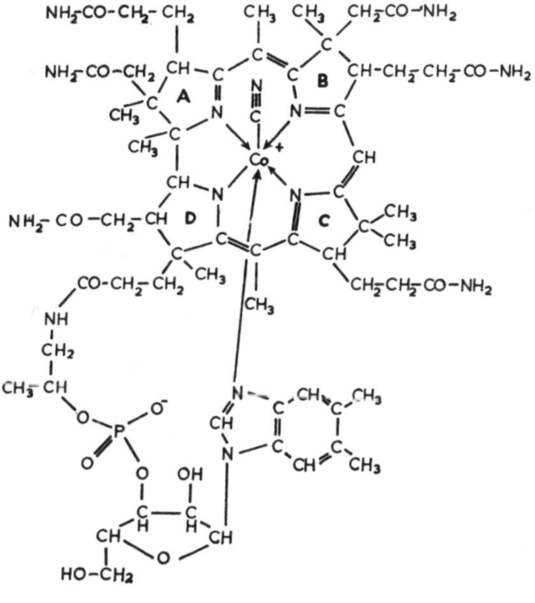

59

Cyanocobalamin; Vitamin B_{12}
(a non-porphyrin member)

APPENDIX

TETRAPYRROLES

BILICHROMES

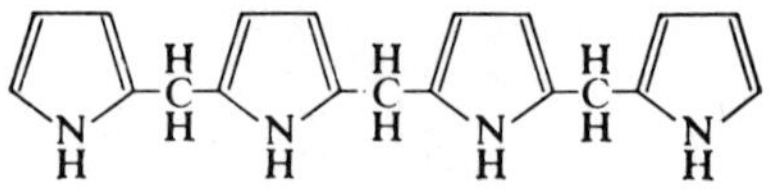

bilane

60

(colorless, not of natural occurrence)

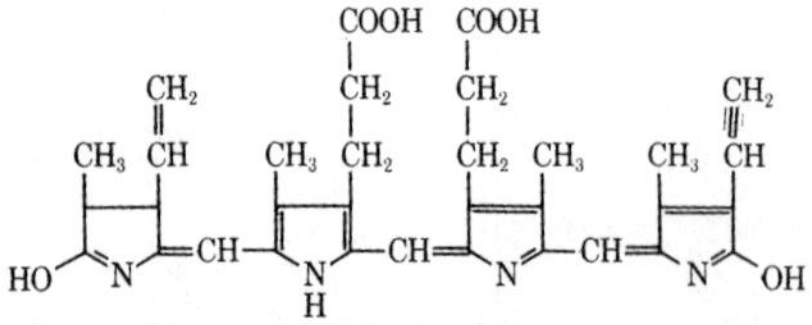

Biliverdin
$C_{33}H_{34}O_6N_4$

61

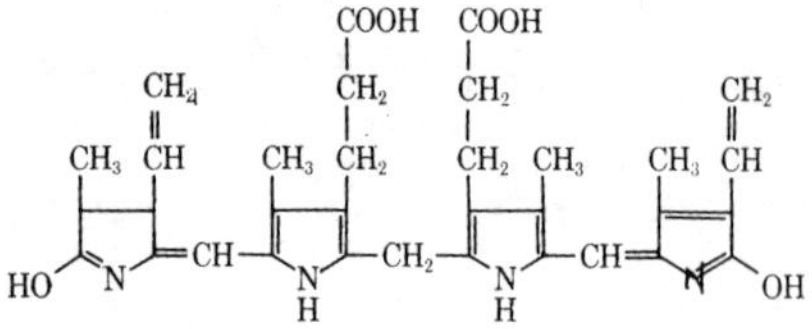

Bilirubin
$C_{33}H_{36}O_6N_4$

62

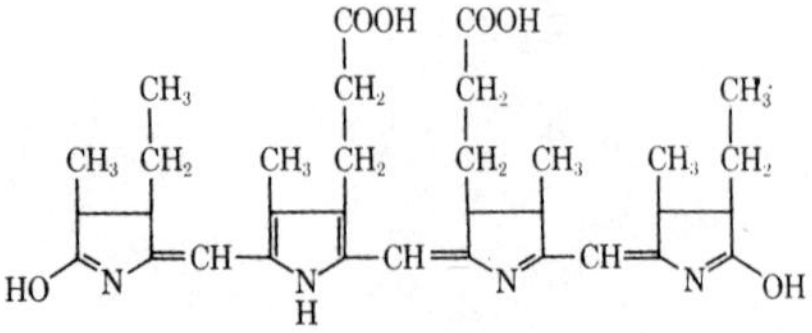

Glaucobilin
$C_{33}H_{38}O_6N_4$

63

BILICHROMES

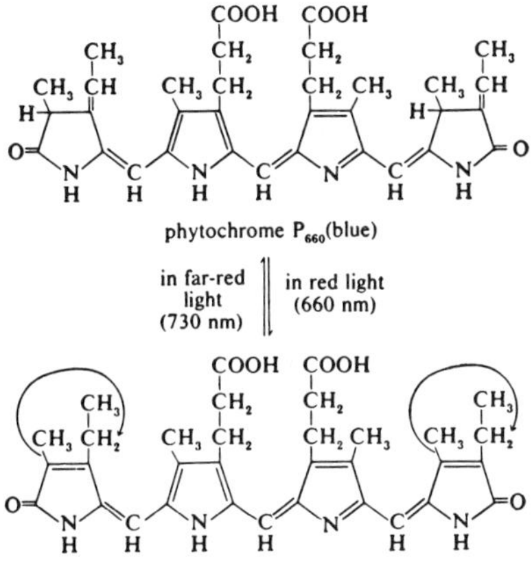

phytochrome P$_{660}$(blue)

in far-red light (730 nm) ‖ in red light (660 nm)

64

phytochrome P$_{730}$

FLAVINE, PURINE, and PTERIN TYPES

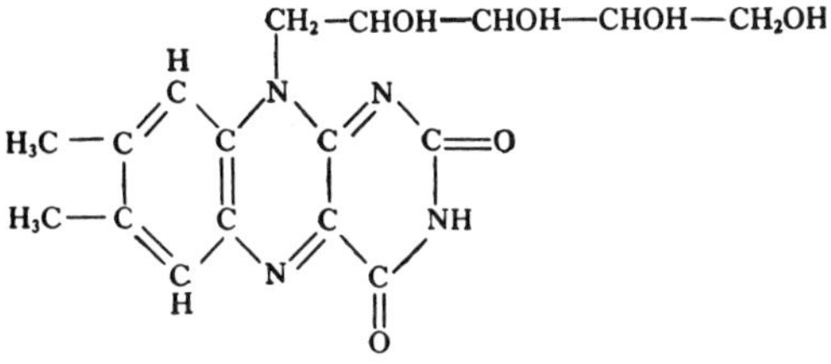

CH$_2$—CHOH—CHOH—CHOH—CH$_2$OH

65

Riboflavin

66a

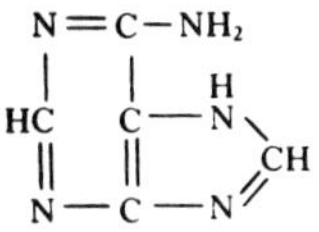

Adenine

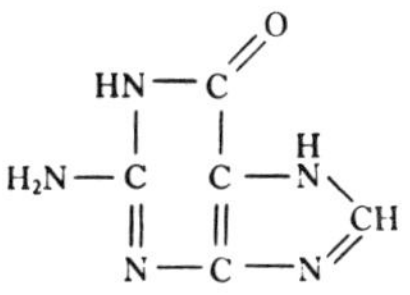

66b

Guanine

Purines

Purines

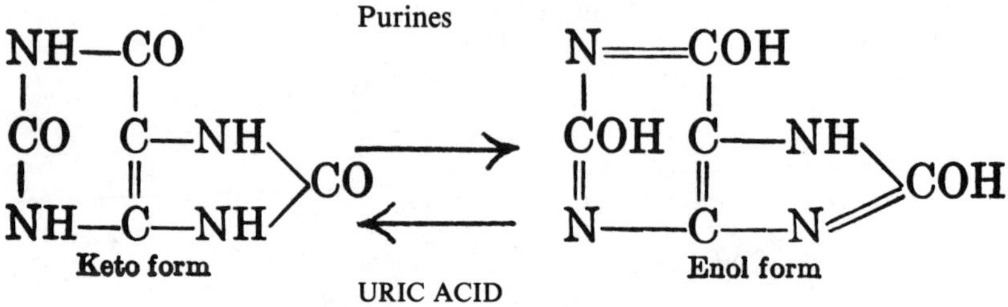

Keto form   Enol form

URIC ACID

67

Tautomeric forms of Uric Acid

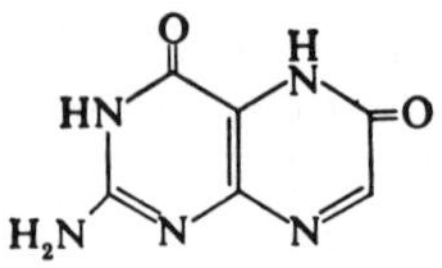

xanthopterin   68

Leukopterin

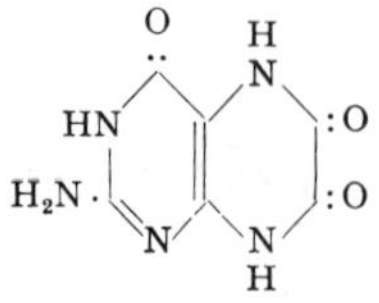

69

Ichthyopterin

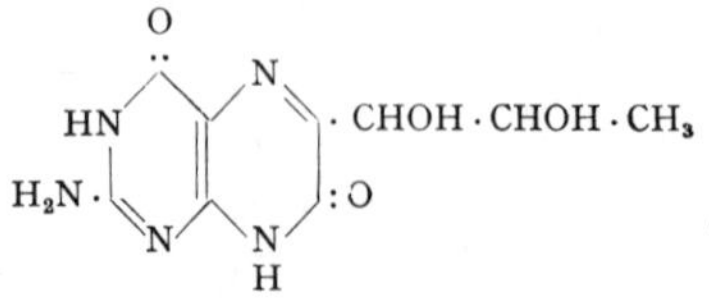

70

Pterins

Selected Bibliography

(for Supplementary Consultation)

Beddard, F. E. (1892). *Animal Coloration. An Account of the Principal Facts and Theories Relating to the Colours and Markings of Animals.* London: Swan Sonnenschein; New York: Macmillan.

Cott, H. B. (1940). *Adaptive Coloration in Animals.* London and New York: Oxford University Press.

Fox, D. L. (1976). *Animal Biochromes and Structural Colours.* Berkeley, Los Angeles, London: University of California Press.

Fox, H. M., and G. Vevers. (1960). *The Nature of Animal Colours.* New York: Macmillan.

Giannasi, D. E., and K. J. Niklas (1977). *Science 197,* 765-767.

Goodwin, T. W. (1954). *Carotenoids. Their Comparative Biochemistry.* New York: Chemical Publishing.

Goodwin, T. W., ed. (1976). *Chemistry and Biochemistry of Plant Pigments.* 2 Vols. London, New York, San Francisco: Academic Press.

Isler, Otto, ed. (1971). *Carotenoids.* Basel and Stuttgart: Birkhäuser-Verlag.

Kennedy, Gilbert Y. et alia multa. (1975). *The Biology and Role of Porphyrins and Related Structures.* Ann. N.Y. Acad. Sci. *244,* 1-700.

Lee, Welton L. (1977). *Carotenoproteins in Animal Coloration.* Stroudsberg, Pa.: Dowden, Hutchinson & Ross.

Lemberg, R., and J. W. Legge. (1949). *Hematin Compounds and Bile Pigments.* New York and London: Interscience.

Mayer, F., and A. H. Cook. (1943). *The Chemistry of Natural Coloring Matters.* New York: Van Nostrand Rheinhold.

Needham, Arthur E. (1974). *The Significance of Zoochromes.* Berlin, Heidelberg; New York: Springer-Verlag.

Newbigin, M. I. (1898). *Colour in Nature.* London: John Murray.

Newton, Sir Isaac (1730). *Opticks.* (Reprinted from the Fourth Edition by Bell & Sons, London, 1931.)

Palmer, L. S. (1922). *Carotinoids and Related Pigments. The Chromolipoids.* New York: Chemical Catalog Co.

Parker, G. H. (1948). *Animal Colour Changes and Their Neurohumours.* London and New York: Cambridge University Press.

Poulton, E. B. (1890). *The Colours of Animals.* London: Kegan Paul, Trench, Trübner.

Rauen, H. M. (1964). *Biochemisches Taschenbuch.* Berlin, Göttingen, and Heidelberg: Springer-Verlag.

Roche, J. (1936). *Essai sur le Biochimie Génerále et Compareé des Pigments Respiratoires.* Paris: Masson.

Rønneberg, H., Gunnar Borch, Denis L. Fox, and Synnøve Liaaen Jensen. *Animal Carotenoids 19.* Alloporin, a new carotenoprotein. *Comp. Biochem. Physiol.* In Press, 1979.

Simon, Hilda (1971). *The Splendor of Iridescence. Structural Colors in the Animal World.* New York: Dodd, Mead.

Verne, J. (1926). *Les Pigments dans l'Organisme Animal.* Paris: Gaston Doin.

Verne, J. (1930). *Coleurs et Pigments des Etres Vivants.* Paris: Librairie Armand Colin.

Verne, J., and F. Layani. (1938). *Les Dyschromies. Traité de Dermatologie.* Paris: Gaston Doin.

Wood, R. W. (1934). *Physical Optics.* New York: Macmillan.

Index

Acacia, plant parasitized by lac insects, 98

Acmaea cassa, A. digitalis, A. scabra, limpets of higher tide levels, rich myoglobin supplies in, 144

Actinia equina (sea anemone), actiniohematin (= hematoporphyrin) in, 151

coloration and carotenoids of, 40

Adamsia palliata (sea anemone), actiniohematin in, 152

Adenine (App. 66a), in nucleic acids, 178

Adenochrome, a red-purple pigment in branchial hearts of *Octopus*, 199-204

chemical properties of, 203-204

microscopic appearance of, *in situ*, 200

probable significance of, 203-204

Adenosine nucleotide, liberation of ammonia from, 178

Aglais urticae (butterfly). *See* Xanthommatin

Ajaia ajaja (roseate spoonbill), pl. 10

carotenoids in plasma and in red cell "ghosts," 79-80

habitat, food gathering and feather pigmentation of, 79

Akara bullata (sea slug), uroporphyrin I in skin of, 154

Albedo, ratio of reflected to incident light intensity: its effects on maintenance of skin carotenoids in opal-eye fish, 69

Algae, carotenoids in, 32-36

iridescence in, 19

Alizarin (App. 34), a red anthraquinone of Madder root and other plants, 99

presence in human bones from a 2000-year burial in Qumran, on the Dead Sea, 99

Alligator mississippiensis, blue-fluorescing pterin in retinal and choroid tissues of, 186

Allopora californica (purple coral, pl. 31), astaxanthin in, chemically linked to protein and to calcium in skeleton of, 39

Ambystoma mexicana (axolotl), skin melanophores of, 115

Amphibians (frogs, toads, salamanders), coloration and carotenoids of, 72-74

Anemia makrinii (fern), iridescence in leaflets of, 19

Anemones. *See* Coelenterates and generic names

Angara calcar, A. lima. See Porphyrins, shell

Conger vulgaris (conger), flavin in melanophoric skin of, 176

Copper proteins of body fluids, 189-195

enzyme members, e.g., tyrosinase, ceruloplasmin and erythrocuprein, 189-190

valence state of copper in, 189-190

Coproporphyrins I and III (App. 58), origins and chemistry of, 148-149

Corals. *See* Coelenterates

Corella parallelogramma. See Ascidians

Cottidae (sculpins), blue-green pigmentation by bilichromes in, 170

Crinoids (sea lilies), paucity of carotenoids in, 48-49

Crop milk of flamingos, red color of, from presence of canthaxanthin, 83

Crotalus terrificus (rattlesnake), xanthophylls, no carotenes or flavins in blood plasma of, 74, 177

Crustaceans, carotenoids of, 57-60

conversion of β-carotene into oxygenated products, e.g., canthaxanthin and astaxanthin by, 59

Ctenosaura hemilopha (spiny iguana), xanthophyllic carotenoid in skin pits of, 75

Cucumaria lacta (sea cucumber), blue ovaries bearing carotenoid protein complex, 48

C. miniata, properties of its hemoglobin, 141

Cura foremanii (flatworm), uroporphyrin in, 150

Cyamon neon (sponge), carotenoids of, 37-38

Cyanocitta (jay), blue plumage of, from Tyndall scattering, 6

Cyanocobalamin. *See* Vitamin B_{12}

Cyclopterus lumpus (lumper or lump-sucker), rich astaxanthin deposits in liver of, 66

Cytochromes (App. 55) as biocatalysts, 4

combined iron in, and function thereof, 128-129

Cytoflav from hog's heart. *See* Riboflavin

Dactylopius coccus, scale insect parasitic on cactus *Nopalea coccinelifera,* source of cochineal dye, 97

D. ceylonicus, source of cochineal dye, 97

Dactylus glomerata (cocksfoot grass), a source of flavone quercitin, eaten by "marbled white" butterfly, 103

Dactynotus, an aphid parasite of plant hosts, 100

Daphnia magna (water flea), a freshwater crustacean

hemoglobin of, concentration variable with conditions, 140

hemoglobin of, high oxygen capacity, 139

Daucus carota (carrot), carotene in, 25-26

Dendraster excentricus (purple sand dollar, pl. 8)

carotenoids in, 47

echinochrome in, 95

D. laevis (smooth or brown sand dollar), unidentified green pigment instead of red or purple echinochrome in, 96

Dendrobates tinctorius (spotted frog), carotenoids in, 73

iron; incapable of oxygen transport, 133

normal occurrence in vertebrate blood at low concentrations, 133

Metridium senile (sea anemone, pl. 27)

actiniohematin in, 151

carotenoid metabolism in, 42-43

color genotypes and carotenoids in, 40-41

melanism in, 111

uric acid from, 178

whiteness of, 8

Microcrustaceans with dissolved (non-cellular) hemoglobin, 139-141

Microgaster conglomeratus (parasitic wasp in caterpillar of white butterfly, *Pieris brassicae*), transfer of host's carotenoids to own cocoon silk, 61-62

Mites, generation of astaxanthin by, 62

Molgula occulta. See Ascidians

Molluscs (bivalves, snails, slugs, cephalopods)

carotenoids in, 50-56

porphyrins in, 154-156

Molpadia intermedia (sea cucumber), properties of hemoglobin of, 141

Mongolian patches of blue skin in infants, 10

Morpho menelaus (butterfly, pl. 2), basis of iridescent blue in wings of, 16

Muroena helena (blenny), skin flavin richness correlated with melanophore concentrations, 177

Mustelus vulgaris (shark), loss of flavin from eggs after fertilization, 175

Myoglobin (see also hemoproteins), in buccal mass of pharyngeal muscles in marine gastropod species, 143-145

Myticola intestinalis (copepod parasitic in mussel), red with hemoglobin; also astaxanthin in females, 51

Mytilus californianus (sea mussel), carotenoids in, 50-51

M. edulis (cosmopolitan bay mussel), carotenoids in, 51

Myxotheca arenigola (foraminiferan protozoan), red colored, 35

Myzus, a parasitic aphid, 100

Naphthoquinones of higher plants and bacteria, recovery in colored, crystalline form, 92

Narwhal, whiteness of skin, 8

Nereis diversicolor (marine polychaete worm), phaeophorbide *a* and coproporphyrin III in gut wall of, 157

Nezaria viridula, N. viridula torquata (herbivorous pentatomid bugs), green wings involving xanthopterin plus a blue bilichromoprotein, 184

Nitrogen fixation catalyzed by hemoglobin in legume root-nodules, 126

Norrisia norisii (red turban snail), immersed resident at low tide levels, has pale store of myoglobin, 145

Notothenia rossi marmorata ("South Georgia Cod"). *See* Icefishes

Ocnius brunneus (sea cucumber), blue carotenoid protein in ovaries of, 48

pod) astaxanthin in, 50

Poison oak dermatitis (via lobinol), treatment with alcoholic ferric chloride, 111

Poisonous skin secretion of some richly pigmented amphibians, 73

Polycheira rufescens (purple holothurian or sea cucumber), naphthoquinone pigment in body wall of, 96

Polycirrus haematoides (polychaete worm), bearing corpuscular hemoglobin, 138

Polyspira, a red protozoan, parasitic in eyes of crustaceans, 35

Pomacea canaliculatus australis (herbivorous freshwater snail), ovorubin, a red astaxanthin glycoprotein in eggs of, 52

Porifera. *See* Sponges

Porphins (App. 54-58, pls. 4, 5, 38-44), 125-164
  chemical structure of, 125-126
  complexed with iron, copper or zinc, 127
  significance in living processes, 126
  synthesized by all organisms, 127

Porphyria diseases, chief types, 131-132

Porphyrins, in ambergris, 161-162
  biological role of, 23
  in birds, 157-161
  character of, 23
  in fishes, 156-157
  as fossils of great geological age, 162-164
  in molluscs, 154-156
  names and chemical structure of, 149-151
  occurrence of in nature, 149-164

in pearls, 156
in porphyria diseases, 128
as primitive biochromes, 26
as series of chlorophyll degradation products in tube worm polychaete *Chaetopterus variopedatus,* 154
in shells of birds' eggs, current and fossilized, 128, 159
stimulation of estrus by, 160-161
in white matter of central nervous system in warm-blooded vertebrates, but lacking in such tissues of cold-bloods, 159-160

Porpita (hydrozoan coelenterate), blue pigment in, 38

Portunus trituberculatus (crab), carotenoid metabolism of, 59

"Port-wine" blemishes. *See* Purple nevus

Potamilla reniformis and *P. stichophthalamos* (marine worms), concentration of melanophores and of flavins in skin of, 177
  hemoglobin in muscle, chlorocruorin in blood of, 143

Prorocentrum micans (marine dinoflagellate), contributor to colored water, 34

Proteins, basis of specific differences, 1

Proteus anguineus (pale, blind cave salamander), carotenoids in tissues of, 72-73

Protoaphin (App. 45), a yellow anthraquinone from black aphis, 100

Protoporphyrin (App. 56), in annelid worms, 154
  chemical structure of, 147-148
  in jellyfish and medusae, 152
  in internal bleeding (feces), 162